GASTRI

MW01114678

COOKBOOK:

MAIN COURSE –
60 Delicious Low-Sugar, Low-Fat,
High Protein Main Course Dishes
for Lifelong Eating Style After
Weight Loss Surgery

Selena Lancaster

Disclaimer

The information contained in this eBook does not
constitute medical advice. Readers who are in need of
medical advice should consult a physician and/or a medical
health professional. Readers who are in need of specific
dietary advice relating to their condition should consult a
dietician and/or a medical health professional.

If you think you are suffering from a medical condition, you
should seek professional health services right away. Do not
delay seeking medical advice, or forego medical advice
already given, because of any information presented in this
eBook .

No warranties are given in relation to the medical
information presented in this eBook. No liability will accrue
to the writer and/or eBook publisher in the event that the
reader and/or user suffers any loss as a result of reliance, in
part or in full, upon the information presented in this
eBook.

Get a BONUS gift exclusive to my readers for FREE!

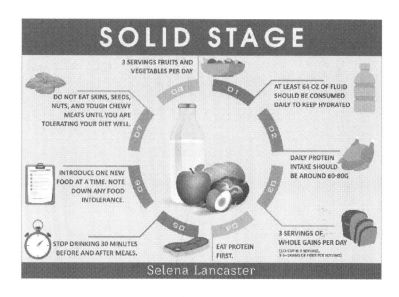

☐ A4-sized printable **Complete Food List Poster** for fluid and puree stages

☐ A4-sized printable Daily **Dietary Reminders Posters** for all post-surgery stages

Scan the QR code and get yours now!

MAIN COURSE
GASTRIC SLEEVE COOKBOOK

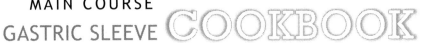

CONTENT

1-11

INTRODUCTION

12-21

TIPS ON FOOD PREPARATION

22-45

POULTRY RECIPES

Chicken Caprese	22
Asian Chicken Lettuce Wrap	24
Chicken Cheesesteak Wrap	26
Turkey Bean Enchilada	28
Portuguese Piri Piri Chicken	30
Garlic Chicken with Mushroom	32
Pan Roasted Chicken With Mediterranean Vegetables	34
Chutney Peppered Turkey Medallions	36
Skinny Chipotle Turkey Meatloaf	38
Thai-Styled BBQ Chicken	40
Tandoori Chicken	42
Slow cooked Salsa Chicken	44

46-69

FISH RECIPES

Scallops with Spicy Papaya Sauce	46
Pan-Fried Rainbow Trout	48
Crunchy Tuna Patties	50
Lemon-Broiled Orange Roughy	52
Baked Tilapia	54
Skinny Fish Sticks	56
Tomato Basil Tilapia	58
Halibut Salad	60
Curry Fish Fillets	62
Grilled Garlic Salmon	64
Cajun Tilapia	66
White Fish and Broccoli Casserole	68

70-93

BEEF RECIPES

Simple Taco Soup	70
Beef and Broccoli Stir Fry	72
Skinny Beef Stroganoff	74
Italian-esque Beef and Veggie Saute	76
Meatloaf Cupcakes With Mashed Cauliflower	78
Garden Vegetable-Beef Soup	80
Beef stuffed Zucchini	82
Indian Beef Madras Curry	84
Elk steaks in mushroom gravy	86
Slow Cooked Round Steak	88
Skinny Bolognese Sauce	90
Southwest Beef with Grilled Peppers	92

94-105

PORK RECIPES

Chinese Pork and Celery Stir Fry	94
Garlic Lime Marinated Pork Chops	96
Mega Pork Meatballs	98
Crustless Quiche	100
Beer-Grilled Pork Chops	102
Skinny Chalupa	104

106-117

LAMB RECIPES

Lemon Mustard Lamb Chop	106
Dijon and Herbs Lamb Chops	108
Lamb Rogan Josh	110
Spicy Lamb Kebab	112
Classic Lamb Stew	114
Braised Lamb Shanks and White Beans	116

118-129

SEAFOOD RECIPES

Shrimp Scampi	118
Shrimp And Shirataki Fettuccine	120
Lemon-Dill Grilled Shrimp	122
Crispy Shrimp With Japanese Cocktail Sauce	124
Shrimp Ceviche	126
Shrimp Jambalaya	128

130-141

VEGETARIAN RECIPES

Creamy Curry Tofu	130
Skinny Mozzarella Sticks	132
Southwest Tofu Scramble	134
Tofu Noodle Alfredo	136
Veggie meatloaf	138
Green Bean and Wisconsin Cheese Casserole	140

Nutrition Summary

POULTRY	Cal (kcal)	Protein (g)	Fat (g)	Carbs (g)	Sugar (g)	Sodium (mg)	Time
Chicken Caprese	153	22.0	4.0	2.7	1.2	70	30 min
Asian Chicken Lettuce Wrap	155	16.0	4.0	11.0	4.0	637	30 min
Chicken Cheesesteak Wrap	156	23.7	4.8	8.9	1.4	271	30 min
Turkey Bean Enchilada	144	11.4	4.8	10.5	0.0	325	40 min
Portuguese-styled Piri Piri Chicken	120	22.2	3.3	1.7	0.6	535	40 min
Garlic Chicken with Mushroom	141	23.8	3.2	1.9	1.1	517	40 min
Pan Roasted Chicken With Mediterranean Vegetables	154	20.0	4.0	9.0	2.0	328	1 hour
Chutney Peppered Turkey Medallions	171	23.1	4.8	5.8	4.2	314	1 hour
Skinny Chipotle Turkey Meatloaf	158	28.2	1.8	7.0	1.6	361	1.5 hours
Thai-Styled Bbq Chicken	178	25.3	3.0	14.5	3.2	263	2.5 hours
Tandoori Chicken	156	24.9	3.1	4.2	3.3	268	6.5 hours
Slow cooked Salsa Chicken	242	38.0	3.3	11.0	2.3	668	8 hours

FISH	Cal (kcal)	Protein (g)	Fat (g)	Carbs (g)	Sugar (g)	Sodium (mg)	Time
Scallops with Spicy Papaya Sauce	172	38.0	4.4	12.5	4.3	346	15 min
Pan-Fried Rainbow Trout	240	25.0	5.0	10.0	0.0	338	20 min
Crunchy Tuna Patties	80	12.0	1.0	4.0	0.0	240	20 min
Lemon-Broiled Orange Roughy	114	17.0	4.0	3.0	0.0	157	20 min
Baked Tilapia	121	20.1	4.3	1.3	0.3	282	20 min
Skinny Fish Sticks	188	26.0	5.0	7.9	0.1	169	25 min
Tomato Basil Tilapia	162	21.4	4.2	4.7	4.4	368	30 min
Halibut Salad	95	13.7	2.1	4.5	3.1	364	30 min
Curried Fish Fillets	191	27.9	3.5	12.0	4.5	292	30 min
Grilled Garlic Salmon	186	17.2	3.5	1.0	0.0	50	35 min
Cajun Tilapia	159	21.0	5.0	1.0	0.0	305	35 min
White Fish And Broccoli Casserole	145	25.6	2.8	4.3	2.0	273	45 min

BEEF	Cal (kcal)	Protein (g)	Fat (g)	Carbs (g)	Sugar (g)	Sodium (mg)	Time
Simple Taco Soup	108	10.0	1.1	14.6	1.4	268	30 min
Beef and Broccoli Stir Fry	119	13.3	4.8	5.5	1.2	159	30 min
Skinny Beef Stroganoff	141	17.4	4.7	6.9	2.5	394	30 min
Italian-esque Beef and Veggie Saute	117	14.4	4.6	4.5	2.4	458	40 min
Meatloaf Cupcakes With Mashed Cauliflower	117	11.9	4.6	6.7	2.4	373	50 min
Garden Vegetable-Beef Soup	122	15.2	3.0	8.7	4.0	510	50 min
Beef stuffed Zucchini	173	18.2	4.8	12.9	3.2	337	1 hour
Indian Beef Madras Curry	160	24.3	4.8	4.9	1.0	389	2 hous
Elk steaks in mushroom gravy	122	16.9	2.3	7.2	2.8	430	5.5 hours
Slow Cooked Round Steak	142	15.8	4.8	8.5	0.9	205	6.5 hours
Skinny Bolognese Sauce	138	14.1	4.4	10.4	4.5	575	6.5 hours
Southwest Beef with Grilled Peppers	176	27.1	4.1	7.7	4.7	292	6.5 hours

PORK	Cal (kcal)	Protein (g)	Fat (g)	Carbs (g)	Sugar (g)	Sodium (mg)	Time
Chinese Pork and Celery Stir Fry	83	12.5	1.9	3.8	1.7	290	30 min
Garlic Lime Marinated Pork Chops	112	19.0	3.0	0.9	0.0	184	40 min
Mega Pork Meatballs	129	13.1	3.8	11.1	3.0	279	40 min
Crustless Quiche	107	18.7	1.4	4.5	1.2	514	1 hour
Beer-Grilled Pork Chops	131	17.8	3.0	5.3	2.0	265	4.5 hours
Skinny Chalupa	124	11.0	3.0	14.0	0.7	184	10 hours

LAMB	Cal (kcal)	Protein (g)	Fat (g)	Carbs (g)	Sugar (g)	Sodium (mg)	Time
Lemon Mustard Lamb Chop	115	17.5	4.2	0.6	0.0	55	30 min
Dijon and Herbs Lamb Chops	134	18.6	4.6	1.2	0.1	320	30 min
Lamb Rogan Josh	138	13.5	4.9	10.0	2.6	369	40 min
Spicy Lamb Kebab	85	14.0	2.4	1.3	0.9	44	3.5 hours
Classic Lamb Stew	174	13.6	4.9	13.2	2.3	87	8.5 hours
Braised Lamb Shanks and White Beans	160	19.2	3.4	12.9	0.0	440	8.5 hours

SEAFOOD	Cal (kcal)	Protein (g)	Fat (g)	Carbs (g)	Sugar (g)	Sodium (mg)	Time
Shrimp Scampi	124	18.1	4.5	2	0.1	310	15 min
Shrimp And Shirataki Fettuccine	158	15.7	4.9	3	0	198	25 min
Lemon-Dill Grilled Shrimp	162.5	33	3.4	3	0	434	25 min
Crispy Shrimp With Japanese Cocktail Sauce	156	33.9	1.4	13.5	0.9	560	25 min
Shrimp Ceviche	160	25	1	13	5	265	25 min
Shrimp Jambalaya	113	15	4.2	7.5	4.2	501	9 hours

VEGETARIAN	Cal (kcal)	Protein (g)	Fat (g)	Carbs (g)	Sugar (g)	Sodium (mg)	Time
Creamy Curry Tofu	139	13.0	4.9	11.8	1.6	363	20 min
Skinny Mozzarella Sticks	93	9.0	4.8	4.1	1.0	243	30 min
Southwest Tofu Scramble	103	10.7	2.2	8.7	0.2	95	30 min
Tofu Noodle Alfredo	144	23.4	4.7	12.5	1.6	562	30 min
Veggie meatloaf	125	10.4	4.6	10.2	1.6	496	55 min
Green Bean and Wisconsin Cheese Casserole	114	7.6	3.6	10.1	2.8	118	1.5 hours

Part I Introduction

About four weeks after your gastric sleeve surgery, your body should be well on its way to recovery, particularly your stomach. If your system has taken well to the fluid, puree and soft food diet stages in the first three weeks after your sleeve gastrectomy, then your surgeon or dietitian can now recommend that you move on to the next phases of the post-surgery diet, which is the solid food stage.

During the puree stage, your stomach should have adjusted to the reintroduction of many common food items in your diet, such as vegetables, fish, chicken, and beef. By this time, you would also be aware that the amount of food you can now intake should be very regulated because your stomach has gotten smaller, which means less food can be consumed. Your goal should now be to get used to consuming nutrient-dense foods which pack more nutrition in smaller amounts, allowing you to get the nourishment your body needs.

In this stage, you will find yourself slowly being able to eat more and more of the foods you normally could consume before gastric sleeve surgery, but it is very important also at this point in time to develop good eating habits that would reinforce your weight loss goals. Remember, gastric sleeve surgery is only one major step in your journey towards a healthier, more fit version of yourself. After sleeve gastrectomy, it is now your responsibility to ensure that what you eat also complements this target.

Taking things slowly but surely, one step at a time, should always be practiced especially as you recover from weight loss surgery. There may be a hankering to immediately return to normalcy and eat foods that are not yet recommended for your condition. If you do this without any regard for your dietitian or surgeon's explicit orders, you are opening up yourself to many post-surgery complications that would further hinder your weight loss goals.

On the third and fourth weeks after your gastric sleeve surgery, the stomach and sleeve are still particularly sensitive, so it is extremely important to always follow the recommendations of your physician or dietitian with regard to what you can and cannot eat, as well as other guidelines on how often to eat, what to observe, etc. Chewing slowly and very thoroughly, for instance, is a very important thing to remember during the soft food stage. This allows the food to be more easily digested by your still-recovering digestive system.

Chewing thoroughly and slowly may, in fact, be a foreign concept to many people who are used to quick, fastfood meals on-the-go. Much of today's lifestyle revolves around easily-microwaved, easily-purchased processed meals that are consumed while driving, walking, and doing other tasks. For so many, chewing food slowly and thoroughly is not a conscious priority and this can lead to many serious health problems later on.

Now that you have undergone sleeve gastrectomy, you will know first-hand how important it is to not only choose your food, but also chew your food. If it is not chewed properly, it can be more difficult for your sleeve and stomach to absorb and digest. Take your time to enjoy the flavors and get yourself used to the process of chewing and swallowing all over again, as you may have gotten so used to just drinking fluids and pureed foods over the previous three weeks.

During the introduction of soft foods into your post-op diet, nausea and vomiting will be avoided if foods are introduced more gradually. The focus will be to consume meals that are high in protein and without too much fat or sugar. Protein is what your body needs at this stage to become stronger, to recover lost energy from the last few weeks, and to help your body achieve optimum balance once again. Fat and sugar, on the other hand, may not be tolerated well by your stomach in high amounts.

Skim milk and protein shakes from your fluid and puree stage are still recommended during the solid food stage while your body is not yet getting enough of its protein requirements from soft and solid foods. Note, however, that any smoothies or fruit shakes should still be monitored for sugar content. Even a seemingly healthy fruit smoothie with too much sugar can irritate your stomach and cause nausea or vomiting, so limit sugar as much as possible.

How much should you eat? Three small meals throughout the day would be recommended by your doctor or dietitian, but healthy snacks throughout the day would likely also be allowed to allow your body to get more nourishment. This is especially true if your body is taking well to the reintroduction of foods at each stage after your gastric sleeve surgery, and if complications or other post-surgery issues have been avoided.

Healthy, highly-nutritious snacks are also important during the solid food stage because they will introduce you to healthier options for snacks which you can adopt for life. Some of these healthy snack items include oatmeal, hard-boiled eggs, bananas, baked sweet potatoes, strawberries, other fresh fruit cups, and hummus with crackers. Even after you have fully recovered from your sleeve gastrectomy, these snack items are more appropriate for your weight loss goals and should be readily available in your pantry or refrigerator instead of potato chips, candy, and Pop Tarts.

One thing to remember about snacks is to not eat too much so that you lose appetite during the main meals. Snacks are only meant to compliment what you eat during your meals, so they should not be too heavy or timed too close to lunch or dinner. In fact, if you are not particularly hungry and can wait until mealtime, it would be more recommended to just wait. Otherwise, if there are some hunger cravings, it is better to go for a light healthy snack.

Another aspect you should continue is good hydration. The body constantly needs water in order for its processes to work smoothly and without any hitches, including the job of digesting your food and speeding up the healing and recovery of your stomach sleeve. Keep yourself hydrated throughout the day and drink water even when you are not particularly feeling thirsty. On the other hand, you would want to avoid drinking too much water a half hour before meals so you will avoid feeling too full by the time you have to eat.

With regard to drinks, sodas and other caffeinated and carbonated beverages should still be avoided during the solid food stage after your gastric sleeve surgery. Sodas and sugary drinks can irritate your stomach, and also make you feel full and bloated right away. Remember that your goal at this stage is to get as much nutrition from whatever limited amount of food you can fit in your stomach, and high-sugar carbonated drinks certainly do not help at this point. Stick to water and freshly squeezed juices, as well as other recommended drinks such as low-sugar smoothies and fruit shakes.

In fact, it would be to your advantage to do away with sodas completely. For one, sodas often contain high amounts of caffeine which is a diuretic, causing dehydration. Many people think they are quenching their thirst when they reach for that bottle of pop, but in reality they are causing the body to lose more water in the process. Water is still the best beverage to drink when you are thirsty.

Another bad effect of drinking soda is the high sugar content, which can lead to serious medical problems such as cardiovascular disease and diabetes. A typical 12-ounce serving of cola would contain up to 3.3 tablespoons of sugar. This amount can raise your blood glucose levels especially if consumed regularly, causing illness. Of course, sodas also are a contributing factor to weight gain, with just one regular can of soda containing up to 3000 extra calories. Even after you have fully recovered, stay away from colas completely in order to attain your weight loss goals.

Once you are in the solid food stage after your gastric sleeve surgery, you will be able to tolerate most of the usual food items already. This stage would normally happen within 5-6 weeks after your sleeve gastrectomy, and would still be under the supervision of your surgeon or dietitian. Within the solid food stage, you should continue the good eating habits and nutritious choices you have developed within the first few weeks after your surgery, including the focus on more fruits and vegetables in your diet, and avoiding high-fat, high-sugar meals and fare.

Your goal is to get a minimum of 60 grams of protein every day from the foods you consume. This would include not just your lean meats, eggs, and vegetables, but also your protein shakes, smoothies, fruit blends, and other supplements you may be taking. Depending on other factors, your doctor may recommend that you consume more or less protein on a daily basis, so follow your physician's recommendation.

The focus of your solid food stage should be on nutrient-dense foods which allow you to eat less but still get the amount of nutrients you need for your daily tasks. Because you have a limited stomach size now, it is up to you to choose carefully what goes into your digestive system, maximizing the space available. This would mean foregoing sodas and other high-sugar drinks and foods because they make you feel full right away, robbing your body of the chance to consume more nutritious fare.

Nutrient-dense foods include the following:

Kale. The benefits of kale have been widely-discussed in recent years, including the high amounts of vitamins, minerals, antioxidants, fiber, and other nutrients contained in this leafy green. A 100-gram serving of kale already gives you plenty of Vitamin B6, magnesium, potassium, calcium, manganese, copper, vitamins A and C, fiber and protein, but only 50 calories, making it perfect for your fitness goals.

Salmon. Most fish available today are nutrient-dense, but salmon packs more for the punch. A 100-gram serving of wild salmon contains all the B-vitamins, potassium, selenium, magnesium, and Omega-3 fatty acids.

Garlic. Many dishes already contain garlic, so it is not very difficult to incorporate more garlic into your eating habits. Not only does garlic add flavor to food, but it is also packed with vitamins C, B1, and B6, selenium, potassium, calcium, copper, and manganese. Garlic helps to regulate blood pressure and lower your cholesterol levels.

Potatoes. Consumed in moderate amounts, potatoes are very nutritious and should be part of your diet long after gastric sleeve surgery. One large potato is packed with vitamin C, most of the B vitamins, potassium, magnesium, copper, manganese, and iron. Potatoes are high in carbohydrates, so they also provide energy.

Blueberries. Fruits are already generally healthy items you should be eating everyday to begin with, but make sure not to leave out blueberries. They contain powerful antioxidant substances such as anthocyanins and phytochemicals, all of help to keep your body disease-free, not to mention lower blood pressure and regulate cholesterol.

Eggs. Eggs are very affordable and easy to buy. They have been unfairly viewed in the past for their high cholesterol content, but research has proven that dietary cholesterol in eggs does not raise bad cholesterol in your blood. On the other hand, there are plenty of benefits you can get from eggs, including protein and high quality fats, vitamins, minerals, and the antioxidants lutein and zeaxanthine, both of which keep the eyes healthy.

These are just some of the more popular and readily-available nutrient-dense foods you can add to your meal plans. There are plenty of other healthy food choices which you will see in the next few sections. The trick is to plan everything accordingly, so you are not stuck thinking what to eat or what to prepare, and then end up just going for whatever is readily available. Most of the time, what you can readily buy is not the healthiest choice either, and this can be a hindrance to your weight loss goals.

The goal after gastric sleeve surgery is to transform your overall eating habits and instill a healthy routine you can stick to for a long time. With the proper guidance and plenty of planning, this can be achieved and allow you to reach your weight loss goals at the right time.

Part II Tips on Food Preparation

The more preparation and planning you put into your meals, the more success you will have in meeting your nutritional goals, staying healthy, and making the right choices towards your weight loss target. The fact is, eating healthy rarely becomes just a simple decision for anyone to observe. Rather, it is a methodical and strategic series of actions that involve many different aspects of daily planning and changes to habits.

A big part of this course of action may be unlearning your previous knowledge and weaning yourself from old habits. Depending on how you were raised, your environment, culture, and other factors, you may already have many preconceived notions and habits regarding food, some of which may not be good for your health. Other eating habits may not have such a detrimental effect but can set you back in your weight loss goals or hinder your recovery especially after your gastric sleeve surgery.

In this regard, a methodical approach to meal planning and food preparation will help to give you a structured, measurable guide towards making those positive changes in your life. Having a set of guidelines to observe will be far easier than just a vague declaration in your mind that you will try to eat healthier, more nutritious meals. Many food items that may seem nutritious may not even be as beneficial as advertised, so planning ahead with the help of recipes and food shopping guides would be advantageous to you.

Another aspect you should greatly consider is the peace of mind in knowing that when you control more of the food preparation process, you have more oversight on hygiene, food safety, ingredients, and other sanitary considerations. We may not like to think about it as much, but meals prepared commercially or in food establishments are not always up to acceptable health and sanitation standards, and for someone like you with a sensitive stomach soon after sleeve gastrectomy, this can pose serious risks.

Food handling and food safety regulations vary depending on where you reside. While there are general guidelines laid out, and agencies which make sure these food handling procedures are observed, it is impossible for any government agency to oversee each establishment at all times of the day. Most rely on spot checks or inspections to maintain or monitor if establishments are following prescribed guidelines, but it may be a different story altogether in between those inspections.

When you prepare your food yourself, you can ensure that food is handled carefully and prepared in the most sanitary way. You will not worry about whether it was cooked properly or if the ingredients used were no longer fresh, or even if the cooking utensils utilized were properly sanitized. This decreases your risk of illnesses or medical issues which may arise from improper food handling and unsafe preparation.

Of course, another advantage of preparing your own meals is being able to make changes to ingredients, taste, flavors, and other components of meals as appropriate for your nutritional goals and weight loss efforts. You may be pleasantly surprised to find out that many of the meals you enjoy and thought could no longer eat because of their content, such as very high fat, trans fats, or sugar can be tweaked accordingly and fit into your diet. Substituting ingredients for healthier options is another excellent advantage of preparing your own meals, giving you room for variety.

Budgeting

It is not a secret to anyone that eating out or ordering in costs more than preparing your own meals at home. This applies whether you live in a small rural community, a quiet suburb, or a busy downtown apartment complex. Purchasing food from commercial establishments will cost you more, but it is often the option people turn to when there is little time or effort to prepare home-cooked meals.

Take some time to assess how much of your monthly budget you are spending towards food at the moment. You should also have a clear idea of the amount of money you will then save if you choose to prepare more of your meals at home rather than buying outside. This also pertains to smaller purchases such as coffee or snacks. A $4 cup of coffee may not seem like much today, for example, but it adds up to about $80 in a month (that is, if you only drink one cup a day, and only on weekdays). Now consider how much you can save if you switch to a healthier, organic or decaffeinated brand of coffee recommended by your physician, and brew it yourself at home.

When you have a detailed meal plan to follow complete with recipes to cook throughout the week, you can more carefully assess how much of your total budget to allocated towards food. This will eliminate unnecessary spending and reduce the extra purchases for items that are not really needed or beneficial to your nutritional goals. With a meal plan, you can stay within your budget and use the savings for other important expenses.

Depending on where you live, you may be able to opt for stores or establishments that offer more savings when you buy wholesale. With meal plans and recipes, you already know beforehand what ingredients you will need, so you can purchase them wholesale and save more. Many stores also offer coupons and other discounts you can avail of, or rewards and points systems for frequent shoppers. All of these perks come with proper planning and preparations.

Shopping wisely

In your area, look for organic products or stores that offer fresh, organic produce. Organic produce such as fruits and vegetables contain fewer pesticides, bioengineered genes, and fertilizers. Organic livestock, meanwhile, would mean these animals are fed only organic feed instead of antibiotics, growth hormones, or other animal by-products. Generally, organic products are better for your health and lower your risk of many medical conditions.

You may need to do some research around your area for the best sources of organic produce. Organic fruits and vegetable are often sold in smaller markets or stores that are close to the farms where they are harvested because preservatives are also avoided, meaning they are always fresh but have a more limited shelf life. This means you are also assured of fresher ingredients in your home-cooked meals, and the flavors are not synthetic.

Many studies have shown that aside from the risks poses by GMOs, pesticides, and other chemicals in traditionally-grown produce and livestock, organic products also contain more of the essential nutrients that your body needs to stay strong and avoid illness. This is especially important after your gastric sleeve surgery because you are recovering from the operation and also trying to maximize the amount of nutrients you will get from a smaller amount of food intake.

Are there small farmer's markets or cooperatives in your area? Talk to the farmers and suppliers and find out their practices used. You may find out a lot about your local farming and livestock community and realize that you can get fresher, more nutritious food items right around the area where you live instead of going to the more commercially-known big box stores where produce and livestock products are often highly processed. At the same time, you will be helping your local economy by buying organic from smaller farms.

Time Management

One of the biggest obstacles for many people who opt to buy food from outside rather than preparing their own meals is time. Many think they are just too busy with work, school, or other responsibilities to set aside time to prepare their own meals at home. In this scenario, time management and schedule efficiency would play a major role and should be the priority if you are really serious about making positive changes in your eating habits.

No matter how hectic you may think your schedule is, you can always find time to set aside for meal preparation if you make changes to your daily routine. For instance, if you usually have the weekends off, you can schedule most of your food shopping on Saturday or Sunday, and then prepare the ingredients so they are ready-to-cook throughout the week. Depending on the recipes you will be including in your meal plans, you may even be able to freeze or store some of the dishes and then just reheat them throughout the week.

Small steps can help cut down the Cooking time. If you already have your fruits sliced the night before, for example, you can just put them in the blender in the morning and have your fruit smoothie ready. The same goes for vegetables and other ingredients you can already put in your lunch container, ready to go in the morning. Even waking up just a half hour earlier than usual may give you enough time to prepare your own breakfast or lunch before you leave the house.

Are there unnecessary things you have gotten used to during the day which you can leave out of your schedule to give you more time to prepare healthier, more nutritious meals at home? If you really assess what you do throughout the day, you will find that you can almost always work out a few minutes to cook or prepare your own lunch or dinner. This may mean going to bed earlier than usual so you can wake up earlier in the morning, but the results will be well worth the additional effort.

Traffic is an everyday reality many people have to take into consideration. If you live in an area where traffic congestion going to or from work or our other tasks can be particularly heavy at certain times of the day, plan ahead so that you know you can still prepare a healthy meal when you get home. If you find that sitting in traffic makes you crave unhealthy food, bring some healthy snacks along such as apples, bananas, or carrot sticks.

Even the simplest changes to your daily routine will free up enough time for you to prepare meals, and there should be no excuse for this to be achieved. If you are really serious about achieving your weight loss goals, becoming healthier, and getting the most out of your recent gastric sleeve surgery, be prepared to take control of more of the food preparation process.

In the next few pages, you will see simple, easy-to-prepare healthy recipes for the solid food stage after your gastric sleeve surgery. These recipes can assist you greatly in developing positive eating habits and meeting your nutritional needs. Take time to learn the ingredients, read the preparation procedures, and also consult with your physician or dietitian regarding which of these meal recipes would be best suited for your body's nutritional requirements.

Best of all, find ways to make food preparation as fun and enjoyable for you, rather than a tiresome chore to get through. How you prepare your food, as well as your mental and emotional mindset, would have a great impact on how your meals are prepared, not to mention your continuing desire to stick to your goals. Stay positive, enjoy the moment, and allow yourself to savour every aspect of the food preparation process, keeping in mind that each step is one closer to your weight loss goals.

Are there family members or friends you can include in the planning, shopping, or meal preparations? You may work alone, but it can definitely be more fun if you have companions with you, especially if they are also conscious about their health and want to make positive eating changes. Form a support system that would keep you accountable for your dietary choices, and allow you to voice out any concerns or struggles you are going through.

MAIN COURSE

CHICKEN CAPRESE

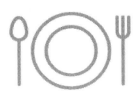

PREP TIME	COOK TIME	SERVES
10 MINUTES	20 MINUTES	6

INGREDENTS

1 pound boneless, skinless chicken breasts

1 tablespoon olive oil

1 teaspoon dry Italian seasoning

4 thick (½-inch) slices ripe tomato

4 1-ounce slices fresh mozzarella cheese

3 tablespoons balsamic vinegar

2 tablespoons thinly sliced basil

Pepper to taste

DIRECTIONS

1. Heat a grill or a grill pan over moderate to moderately high heat.

2. Lightly pour 1 tablespoon of olive oil over chicken breasts and season to taste with pepper.

3. Sprinkle Italian seasoning over the chicken.

4. Place the chicken on the grill and cook for 3 to 5 minutes each side, or until cooked well. Cooking time will vary based on the thickness of your chicken breasts.

5. When chicken is cooked well, top with a slice of mozzarella cheese and cook for an additional minute to two minutes.

6. Remove from heat and place chicken breasts on a separate plate. Top each breast with one slice of tomato, thinly sliced basil and pepper to taste.

7. Season with balsamic vinegar or balsamic glaze and serve.

NUTRITION FACTS (PER SERVING)

CALORIES	153	KCal
PROTEIN	22.0	g
FAT	4.0	g
CARBOHYDRATES	2.7	g
SUGAR	1.2	g
SODIUM	70	mg

MAIN COURSE

ASIAN CHICKEN LETTUCE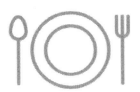

PREP TIME	COOK TIME	SERVES
10 MINUTES	20 MINUTES	4

INGREDENTS

1/2 pound ground chicken breast

1 8-ounce can of bamboo shoots, drained and minced

1 8-ounce can of water chestnuts, drained and minced

8 small leaves butter lettuce

1 whole green onion, chopped

1 small cucumber, seeded and sliced

1 cup minced onion

3 tablespoons sherry cooking wine

2 tablespoons hoisin sauce

1 tablespoon unsalted peanut butter

2 teaspoons low-sodium soy sauce

2 teaspoons hot pepper sauce

2 packets (.035 ounce each) sugar substitute

1 tablespoon minced garlic

1 teaspoon minced ginger

1 teaspoon toasted sesame oil

DIRECTIONS

1. In a medium-sized bowl, combine the bamboo shoots, water chestnuts, sherry, hoisin sauce, peanut butter, soy sauce, hot-pepper sauce, and sugar substitute. Mix well and then set aside.

2. Sauté the onion for 4 minutes or until the onions are fragrant and softened (not too brown).

3. Add the garlic and cook for an additional minute. Increase the heat to medium-high and add the ground chicken, ginger, and salt.

4. Cook the chicken and break into pieces using a spatula or wooden spoon, for 3 to 4 minutes, until no longer pink. Add the bamboo shoot and water chestnut mixture. Cook for 2 minutes, or until heated through. Add the toasted sesame oil and stir well.

5. Remove the pan from the heat. To serve, divide the chicken mixture evening onto each of the 8 lettuce leaves. Top with chopped green onion and cucumber. Serve immediately.

NUTRITION FACTS (PER SERVING)

CALORIES	155	KCal
PROTEIN	16.0	g
FAT	4.0	g
CARBOHYDRATES	11.0	g
SUGAR	4.0	g
SODIUM	637	mg

MAIN COURSE
CHICKEN CHEESESTEAK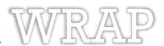

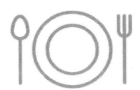

PREP TIME	COOK TIME	SERVES
10 MINUTES	20 MINUTES	2

INGREDENTS

6 ounces boneless, skinless chicken breast, trimmed of visible fat

1/4 cup onions, chopped

1/4 cup green pepper, sliced

1/4 cup mushrooms, sliced

3/4 ounce light swiss cheese

1 whole wheat flour, low-carb tortilla

DIRECTIONS

1. Place chicken breast on cutting board, pound to 1/4" thin and slice into very thin strips.

2. Place a skillet over moderately high heat and mist with cooking spray.

3. Add the onion and chicken to the heated pan and cook until onions are translucent and chicken is no longer pink on all sides.

4. Add green peppers and mushrooms to the pan and cook until peppers and mushrooms soften.

5. Place tortilla between 2 damp paper towels. Microwave for about 20-25 seconds.

6. Lay the warm tortilla flat and spread cheese in an even strip down the middle.

7. Add the chicken, peppers, onions and mushrooms. You may also use chili peppers (optional).

8. Fold sides of tortilla over middle. Serve immediately.

NUTRITION FACTS (PER SERVING)

CALORIES	156	KCal
PROTEIN	23.7	g
FAT	4.8	g
CARBOHYDRATES	8.9	g
SUGAR	1.4	g
SODIUM	271	mg

MAIN COURSE
TURKEY BEAN ENCHILADA

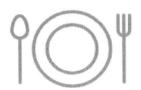

PREP TIME
10 MINUTES

COOK TIME
30 MINUTES

SERVES
8

INGREDENTS

6 medium scallions, white and green parts chopped

12 ounces 93% ground turkey. Sautéed until slightly brown.

12 ounces canned low sodium pinto beans, drained and rinsed

1 cup canned enchilada sauce, divided

4 medium-sized low-carb tortillas

1/4 cup shredded reduced fat Mexican cheese

DIRECTIONS

1. Preheat oven to 350 degrees.

2. Mix scallions, turkey, beans, and ½ cup enchilada or taco sauce.

3. Fill each tortilla with ¼ of turkey-bean mixture. Fold in sides, top and bottom of tortilla to completely enclose the filling inside the tortilla.

4. Place tortillas seam side down in a 9x13-inch baking dish.

5. Pour the remaining ½ cup of sauce over top of enchiladas and add the cheese.

6. Cover pan and bake until heated through and cheese is hot and bubbly (about 20 minutes).

NUTRITION FACTS (PER SERVING)

CALORIES	144	KCal
PROTEIN	11.4	g
FAT	4.8	g
CARBOHYDRATES	10.5	g
SUGAR	0	g
SODIUM	325	mg

MAIN COURSE

PORTUGESE-STYLED
PIRI PIRI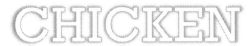

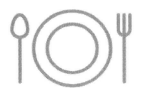

PREP TIME	COOK TIME	SERVES
10 MINUTES	30 MINUTES	4

INGREDENTS

1 pound boneless, skinless chicken breasts

1/4 cup apple cider vinegar

1/2 lemon, juice only

1/2 lime

2 cloves garlic, minced

2 teaspoons chilies, crushed

1 teaspoon oregano

1 teaspoon paprika

1/2 teaspoon salt

1/4 teaspoon pepper

1/4 teaspoon salt

DIRECTIONS

1. In a large bowl, mix together chicken, vinegar, lemon juice, garlic, chilies and all spices. Put it in the fridge to marinate overnight.

2. Preheat the griddle to medium heat. Spray the surface well with non-stick cooking spray.

3. Lay the chicken breast on the griddle and allow to cook for 10 minutes. Flip and cook for another 10-15 minutes until cooked through.

4. Squeeze the lime juice on top on the chicken and serve immediately.

NUTRITION FACTS (PER SERVING)

CALORIES	120	KCal
PROTEIN	22.2	g
FAT	3.3	g
CARBOHYDRATES	1.7	g
SUGAR	0.6	g
SODIUM	535	mg

MAIN COURSE

GARLIC CHICKEN

WITH MUSHROOM

PREP TIME

5 MINUTES

COOK TIME

35 MINUTES

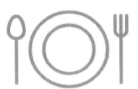

SERVES

4

INGREDENTS

1 pound boneless, skinless chicken breasts

1/2 pound sliced Cremini mushrooms

15 cloves garlic, peeled

1 teaspoon pepper

1/2 teaspoon salt

DIRECTIONS

1. Pre-heat the oven to 375°F

2. Use a kitchen hammer to flatten the chicken breast. Season with salt and pepper

3. Place the chicken in a baking dish and put the mushrooms and garlic on top.

4. Bake for 30 minutes. Wait for 2-3 minutes then serve.

NUTRITION FACTS (PER SERVING)

CALORIES	141	KCal
PROTEIN	23.8	g
FAT	3.2	g
CARBOHYDRATES	1.9	g
SUGAR	1.1	g
SODIUM	517	mg

MAIN COURSE

PAN ROASTED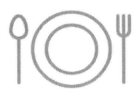

WITH MEDITTERANEAN VEGETABLES

PREP TIME	COOK TIME	SERVES
10 MINUTES	50 MINUTES	8

INGREDENTS

1 medium red onion, peeled and cut into wedges

1 medium zucchini, cut into bite-sized pieces

1 medium yellow pepper, seeded and cut into chunks

1 medium red pepper, seeded and cut into chunks

1 medium eggplant, cut into chunks

8 small chicken thighs, skin removed

3/4 cup low fat, low sodium chicken broth

1/4 cup low-fat and low-sugar tomato pasta sauce or crushed tomatoes 1/4 teaspoon salt

3 tablespoons low-sodium soy sauce

1 tablespoon chopped fresh thyme

DIRECTIONS

1. Preheat the oven to 350 F.

2. Place the onion, zucchini, peppers and eggplant in a large non-stick roasting pan. Spray with low-fat cooking oil or spray to coat on all sides.

3. Place the chicken thighs between the vegetables and sprinkle with the thyme. Roast for about a half hour, turning the chicken thighs every few minutes to make sure all sides are evenly-cooked.

4. Mix the soy sauce, chicken broth and sauce or crushed tomatoes in another container, then pour into the pan over the vegetables and around the chicken pieces.

5. Return to the oven for a further 15-20 minutes or until the chicken is cooked well and the vegetables are tender.

NUTRITION FACTS (PER SERVING)

CALORIES	154	KCal
PROTEIN	20.0	g
FAT	4.0	g
CARBOHYDRATES	9.0	g
SUGAR	2.0	g
SODIUM	328	mg

MAIN COURSE

CHUTNEY PEPPERED

TURKEY MEDALLION

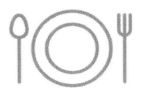

PREP TIME	COOK TIME	SERVES
35 MINUTES	25 MINUTES	4

INGREDENTS

1 pound turkey tenderloins, cut into 3/4-inch strips

1/4 cup low-sodium turkey broth

1/8 cup mango chutney

2 tablespoons brandy

2 tablespoons mixed peppercorns

2 tablespoons green onion, minced

1 1/2 teaspoons olive oil, divided

DIRECTIONS

1. Grind peppercorns and cover the turkey strips fully with the ground pepper. Refrigerate 30 minutes.

2. In a non-stick skillet, sauté turkey in half of the oil over medium heat for 5 minutes per side until cooked through.

3. Sauté onion in the rest of the oil for 30 seconds. Add in broth and brandy. Cook for 2 minutes then turn to low heat and add in chutney.

4. Pour the chutney sauce over the turkey and serve.

NUTRITION FACTS (PER SERVING)

CALORIES	171	KCal
PROTEIN	23.1	g
FAT	4.8	g
CARBOHYDRATES	5.8	g
SUGAR	4.2	g
SODIUM	314	mg

MAIN COURSE

SKINNY CHIPOTLE

TURKEY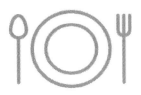

PREP TIME	COOK TIME	SERVES
15 MINUTES	75 MINUTES	8

INGREDENTS

Main Ingredients

1 pound 93% ground turkey

2 Chipotle chillies in adobo sauce (from 7-ounce can), chopped

1/2 cup finely chopped onion

1/2 cup finely chopped zucchini

1/4 cup oatmeal

1/4 cup whole wheat breadcrumbs

1/4 cup low-sodium tomato sauce

2 large egg whites

3 cloves garlic, minced

Spices

2 teaspoons dried parsley

1/2 teaspoon salt

1/2 teaspoon ground cumin

1/2 teaspoon dried oregano

1/4 teaspoon basil

1/4 teaspoon pepper

Toppings

1/4 cup low-sodium tomato sauce

1 tablespoon low sugar/salt ketchup

1/2 teaspoon hot sauce

38

DIRECTIONS

1. Pre-heat the oven to 350 °F.

2. In a large bowl, combine all main ingredients and spices to a uniform consistency.

3. Coat a 9 x 5-inch loaf pan with cooking spray. Pour the mixture into the pan and spread evenly. Bake for 30 minutes

4. Combine all topping ingredients and cover the meatloaf with the sauce evenly. Cover and bake for an extra 30 minutes. Wait for 10 minutes before cutting into 8 mini meatloaf.

NUTRITION FACTS (PER SERVING)

CALORIES	158	KCal
PROTEIN	28.2	g
FAT	1.8	g
CARBOHYDRATES	7.0	g
SUGAR	1.6	g
SODIUM	361	mg

MAIN COURSE
THAI-STYLED BBQ CHICKEN

PREP TIME

2 HOURS

COOK TIME

30 MINUTES

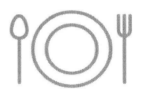

SERVES

4

INGREDENTS

1 pound boneless, skinless chicken breasts

6 ounces fat-free plain yogurt

5 cloves garlic

1 stick lemongrass, chopped

1 1/2 teaspoons black peppercorns

1 1/2 teaspoons stevia, brown sugar blend

1 teaspoon ground turmeric

1 bunch coriander roots

DIRECTIONS

1. Blend lemongrass, garlic, pepper, stevia, turmeric, coriander and 2 tablespoons of yogurt to a smooth consistency.

2. Add the remaining yogurt and blend briefly until just incorporated.

3. In a large bowl, mix the chicken in the sauce until the chicken is covered well. Marinate for 2 hours.

4. Cook on a grill until done.

NUTRITION FACTS (PER SERVING)

CALORIES	178	KCal
PROTEIN	25.3	g
FAT	3.0	g
CARBOHYDRATES	14.5	g
SUGAR	3.2	g
SODIUM	263	mg

MAIN COURSE
TANDOORI CHICKEN

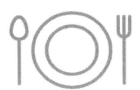

PREP TIME

6 HOURS

COOK TIME

30 MINUTES

SERVES

4

INGREDENTS

14 ounces boneless, skinless chicken breasts

1 cup fat-free plain yogurt

3 tablespoons Tandoori spice mix

2 teaspoons grated fresh ginger

1 teaspoon cumin

DIRECTIONS

1. Mix the chicken in the sauce until the chicken is covered well. Refrigerate overnight.

2. Before cooking, scrap off the sauce. Grill each side for 2 minutes on high heat followed by 5 minutes on each side over low-medium heat.

3. Heat the sauce and pour over the chicken and serve.

NUTRITION FACTS (PER SERVING)

CALORIES	156	KCal
PROTEIN	24.9	g
FAT	3.1	g
CARBOHYDRATES	4.2	g
SUGAR	3.3	g
SODIUM	268	mg

MAIN COURSE

SLOW COOKED
SALSA CHICKEN

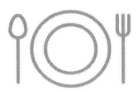

PREP TIME

5 MINUTES

COOK TIME

8 HOURS

SERVES

6

INGREDENTS

1 pound boneless, skinless chicken breasts

1 can 10.5-ounces low-fat cream of mushroom soup

1 cup salsa

1/2 cup low-fat sour cream

1 package low-sodium taco seasoning

DIRECTIONS

1. Place the chicken in the slow cooker

2. Cover the chicken with taco seasoning.

3. Add salsa and soup and mix well.

4. Cook on low for 7-8 hours until desired tenderness.

5. Add in sour cream. Mix well and serve.

NUTRITION FACTS (PER SERVING)

CALORIES	242	KCal
PROTEIN	38.0	g
FAT	3.3	g
CARBOHYDRATES	11.0	g
SUGAR	2.3	g
SODIUM	668	mg

MAIN COURSE

SEARED SCALLOPS

WITH SPICY PAPAYA SAUCE

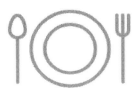

PREP TIME	COOK TIME	SERVES
5 MINUTES	10 MINUTES	4

INGREDENTS

1 **pound** sea scallops

1 small papaya, peeled, seeded and chopped

1 red bell pepper, chopped

1/2 red onion, chopped

2 **tablespoons** all-purpose flour

2 **tablespoons** fresh lime juice

1 **tablespoon** chopped cilantro

1 **tablespoon** olive oil

1 **teaspoon** minced jalapeño peppers

1 **dash** of salt

1 **dash** of pepper

DIRECTIONS

1. Blend papaya, bell pepper, onion, lime juice, cilantro and jalapeño briefly to remove large chunks.

2. In another bowl, mix scallops, flour, salt and pepper evenly. Over medium heat, cook the scallops until golden.

3. Serve the scallops on the papaya sauce.

NUTRITION FACTS (PER SERVING)

CALORIES	172	KCal
PROTEIN	38.0	g
FAT	4.4	g
CARBOHYDRATES	12.5	g
SUGAR	4.3	g
SODIUM	346	mg

MAIN COURSE

PAN FRIED
RAINBOW TROUT

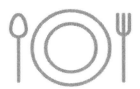

PREP TIME	COOK TIME	SERVES
5 MINUTES	15 MINUTES	2

INGREDENTS

8 ounces rainbow trout fillets

3 tablespoons yellow cornmeal

1 1/3 tablespoon chopped parsley

1/4 teaspoon ground celery seeds

1/4 teaspoon ground black pepper

pinch salt

2 teaspoon olive oil

48

DIRECTIONS

1. Clean and rinse fish fillets. Check to make sure that all bones are removed. Pat dry.

2. In a separate container, mix the cornmeal, salt, pepper, celery seed and chopped parsley.

3. Cover fish with cornmeal mixture and press onto fish fillets.

4. Heat olive oil in non-stick skillet. Cook fish 2 to 3 minutes per side. Fish should be brown and crisp and should flake when pierced with a fork or a knife.

NUTRITION FACTS (PER SERVING)

CALORIES	240	KCal
PROTEIN	25.0	g
FAT	4.9	g
CARBOHYDRATES	10.0	g
SUGAR	0	g
SODIUM	338	mg

MAIN COURSE

CRUNCHY
TUNA PATTIES

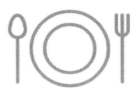

PREP TIME	COOK TIME	SERVES
5 MINUTES	15 MINUTES	8

INGREDENTS

4 3-ounce cans tuna, in water

4 egg whites

16 Wheat Thins crackers, crushed

1/4 cup grated carrot

1/4 cup chopped water chestnuts, capers or diced red pepper

1 tablespoon minced onion, if tolerated

Pepper, dill and dried mustard, to taste

DIRECTIONS

1. Mix all the ingredients together in a container.

2. Form mixture into eight patties with hands.

3. Spray medium-sized skillet with nonstick cooking spray and place over medium heat.

4. Cook patties until golden brown on both sides, 2-3 minutes per side.

NUTRITION FACTS (PER SERVING)

CALORIES	80	KCal
PROTEIN	12.0	g
FAT	1.0	g
CARBOHYDRATES	4.0	g
SUGAR	0	g
SODIUM	240	mg

MAIN COURSE

LEMON-BROILED
ORANGE ROUGHY

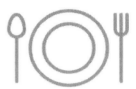

PREP TIME	COOK TIME	SERVES
5 MINUTES	15 MINUTES	4

INGREDENTS

1 pound orange roughy fillets (4 ounces each)

8 medium lemon wedges

3 tablespoons lemon juice

1 tablespoon Dijon mustard

1 tablespoon olive oil

1/4 teaspoon ground pepper

DIRECTIONS

1. Cover the rack of a broiler pan or a baking sheet with tin foil and spray foil with cooking spray.

2. Combine lemon juice, mustard, olive oil and ground pepper. Stir thoroughly.

3. Place fish fillets on rack or baking sheet. Brush fillets with half the lemon juice mixture, and then set aside the remaining half.

4. Broil fish for 5 minutes or until fish flakes easily.

5. Drizzle the remaining lemon juice mixture over the fillets and add pepper.

6. Serve with lemon wedges.

NUTRITION FACTS (PER SERVING)

CALORIES	114	KCal
PROTEIN	17.0	g
FAT	4.0	g
CARBOHYDRATES	3.0	g
SUGAR	0.0	g
SODIUM	157	mg

MAIN COURSE
BAKED TILAPIA

PREP TIME

5 MINUTES

COOK TIME

15 MINUTES

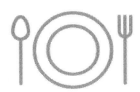

SERVES

1

INGREDENTS

1 tilapia fillet (4 ounces)

1/2 tablespoon lemon juice

1/2 tablespoon reduced fat or light mayonnaise

3/4 tablespoon finely chopped green onions

1/4 teaspoon dried basil

Pinch of salt

Pinch of Black pepper

DIRECTIONS

1. Preheat oven to 350 degrees Fahrenheit.

2. Place the fillet in a buttered baking dish.

3. Sprinkle the top with lemon juice.

4. Bake fish in preheated oven 10 to 20 minutes or until fish starts to flake.

5. Meanwhile, mix the mayonnaise, onions and seasonings in a bowl using a fork.

6. When the fish is ready, spread the top with the mixture and bake until golden brown (approximately 5 minutes, depending on the thickness of the fish).

NUTRITION FACTS (PER SERVING)

CALORIES	121	KCal
PROTEIN	20.1	g
FAT	4.3	g
CARBOHYDRATES	1.3	g
SUGAR	0.3	g
SODIUM	282	mg

MAIN COURSE
SKINNY FISH STICKS

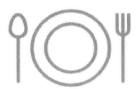

PREP TIME
10 MINUTES

COOK TIME
15 MINUTES

SERVES
4

INGREDENTS

1 **pound** fish fillets

1 large egg

1/3 cup whole-wheat
breadcrumbs

1/4 cup grated Parmesan
cheese

1/2 teaspoon dried
parsley

1/2 teaspoon paprika

1/2 tablespoon light
butter, melted

DIRECTIONS

1. Preheat oven to 450 degrees.

2. In a smaller dish, beat the egg. In a separate dish, combine the bread crumbs, Parmesan cheese, paprika and parsley.

3. Cut the fish into strips, 3 inches long & 1/2 inches wide.

4. Dip each strip into the egg, then into the crumb mixture.

5. Place the fish strips on a lightly greased baking sheet.

6. Drizzle the melted butter over the fish.

7. Bake for 7-10 minutes, or until fish flakes easily with a fork or knife.

NUTRITION FACTS (PER SERVING)

CALORIES	188	KCal
PROTEIN	26.0	g
FAT	4.9	g
CARBOHYDRATES	7.9	g
SUGAR	0.1	g
SODIUM	169	mg

MAIN COURSE
TOMATO BASIL TILAPIA

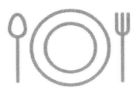

PREP TIME	COOK TIME	SERVES
5 MINUTES	25 MINUTES	4

INGREDENTS

1 **pound** tilapia fillet

1/2 **pound** cherry tomatoes

1/2 **cup** loosely packed fresh basil leaves, torn into halves and thirds, divided

12 garlic cloves, peeled

1/2 **tablespoon** extra virgin olive oil

1/2 **teaspoon** salt

1/4 **teaspoon** pepper

DIRECTIONS

1. Preheat oven to 425 degrees.

2. In a 9 x 13-inch pan, mix the tomatoes, oil, garlic, salt, pepper, and ½ of the basil. Stir well.

3. Roast for 15 minutes, then remove from oven and stir gently for a few seconds.

4. Place the fish fillets in pan with the cherry tomatoes.

5. Place back in oven and continue roasting for another 7 to 10 minutes, or until fish is no longer translucent and tomatoes are juicier.

6. Remove from oven. Divide fish on to individual serving plates.

7. Add the remaining basil leaves to the tomatoes and sprinkle over fish fillets.

NUTRITION FACTS (PER SERVING)

CALORIES	162	KCal
PROTEIN	21.4	g
FAT	4.2	g
CARBOHYDRATES	4.7	g
SUGAR	4.4	g
SODIUM	368	mg

MAIN COURSE
HALIBUT SALAD

PREP TIME

5 MINUTES

COOK TIME

25 MINUTES

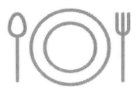

SERVES

4

INGREDENTS

4 cups shredded halibut

1 cup fat-free mayonnaise

1/4 cup chopped green onion

1/4 cup chopped white onion

1/2 cup dill pickle relish

DIRECTIONS

1. In a pot, blanch the halibut until cooked through. Set aside to cool.

2. Use a pair of fork shred the halibut

3. In a large bowl, combine all ingredient. Refrigerate for 15 minutes and serve

NUTRITION FACTS (PER SERVING)

CALORIES	95	KCal
PROTEIN	13.7	g
FAT	2.1	g
CARBOHYDRATES	4.5	g
SUGAR	3.1	g
SODIUM	364	mg

MAIN COURSE
CURRY FISH FILLET

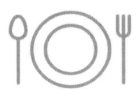

PREP TIME

5 MINUTES

COOK TIME

25 MINUTES

SERVES

5

INGREDENTS

17 1/2 ounces fish fillets

2 large onions, sliced

1/2 green bell pepper, sliced

1/2 red bell pepper, sliced

2 cloves garlic, crushed

1 tablespoon oat bran

1 tablespoon curry powder

1 teaspoon ground cumin seeds

1 teaspoon tomato juice

1 bacon stock cube

1 cup water

Pinch of black pepper

DIRECTIONS

1. Add onions, bell pepper, garlic and tomato juice to a non-stick pan. Simmer over low heat for 5 minutes.

2. Add curry powder, oat bran and cumin while stirring. Break stock cube into smaller pieces in water and add to the mixture. Simmer to a thick consistency.

3. Place the fish fillet in the pan and cooked for 5 minutes. Sprinkle with black pepper and serve.

NUTRITION FACTS (PER SERVING)

CALORIES	191	KCal
PROTEIN	27.9	g
FAT	3.5	g
CARBOHYDRATES	12.0	g
SUGAR	4.5	g
SODIUM	292	mg

MAIN COURSE
GRILLED GARLIC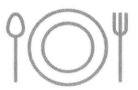

PREP TIME	COOK TIME	SERVES
5 MINUTES	30 MINUTES	4

INGREDENTS

1 large salmon fillet, pan-sized

1/2 **cup** skim milk

3 cloves garlic

1 **teaspoon** lemon pepper

1/2 teaspoon garlic salt

DIRECTIONS

1. Rinse fillet with 1/2 cup milk. To remove fishy odor or taste, you can let it set in milk for up to 5 minutes. Preheat oven to 350 degrees.

2. Spray a skillet. Add in minced garlic.

3. Place in fish, skin side down, and brown for 1 minute. Dust flesh side of fish with garlic salt and lemon pepper. Flip and brown for another minute.

4. Place fish skin side down in pan, transfer entire pan to oven pre-heated at 350 degrees.

5. Roast for 5 minutes per inch of fillet thickness for medium-cooked fish, and 10 minutes per inch for well-done fish.

NUTRITION FACTS (PER SERVING)

CALORIES	186	KCal
PROTEIN	17.1	g
FAT	3.5	g
CARBOHYDRATES	0.9	g
SUGAR	0	g
SODIUM	50	mg

MAIN COURSE
CAJUN TILAPIA

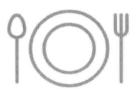

PREP TIME	COOK TIME	SERVES
5 MINUTES	30 MINUTES	4

INGREDENTS

4 (6 ounce) tilapia fillets

1 **tablespoon** unsalted butter

2 **teaspoons** paprika

1 **teaspoon** black pepper

1 **teaspoon** dried thyme

1 **teaspoon** dried oregano

1/2 **teaspoon** garlic salt

1/4 **teaspoon** cayenne pepper

DIRECTIONS

1. Preheat oven to 400 degrees Fahrenheit.

2. Sprinkle all spices and herbs over 3 thawed fish fillets.

3. Place the fish fillets on a non-stick baking sheet.

4. Spread the butter on each fish fillet.

5. Cover the entire pan with aluminium foil and set to bake for approximately 25 minutes or until the fish fillets are flaky.

NUTRITION FACTS (PER SERVING)

CALORIES	168	KCal
PROTEIN	21.0	g
FAT	6.0	g
CARBOHYDRATES	<1	g
SUGAR	0	g
SODIUM	305	mg

MAIN COURSE

WHITE FISH AND
BROCCOLI CASSEROLE

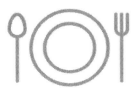

PREP TIME

5 MINUTES

COOK TIME

40 MINUTES

SERVES

6

INGREDENTS

1 pound white fish, or about 6 fillets

10 ounces frozen Broccoli, thawed

1 cup canned mushrooms

1/2 cup Finely Shredded Low-Moisture Part
Skim Mozzarella cheese

Salt and pepper

DIRECTIONS

1. Layer the broccoli in the bottom of a sprayed baking dish, then spread the mushrooms on top of the broccoli.

2. Place the seasoned fish on top of the mushrooms. Sprinkle generously with mozzarella cheese.

3. Bake the fish fillets at 350 degrees for 35 minutes or until the fillets are crispy or flaky.

NUTRITION FACTS (PER SERVING)

CALORIES	145	KCal
PROTEIN	25.6	g
FAT	2.8	g
CARBOHYDRATES	4.3	g
SUGAR	2.0	g
SODIUM	273	mg

MAIN COURSE

SIMPLE TACO BEAN SOUP

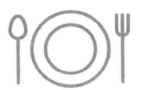

PREP TIME
5 MINUTES

COOK TIME
25 MINUTES

SERVES
24

INGREDENTS

1 **pound** 95% lean ground
beef

1 **package** of taco
seasoning

1.5 ounces fat-free ranch
dressing

2 10.5-ounce **cans** kidney
beans, undrained

2 10.5-ounce **cans** pinto
beans, undrained

2 10.5-ounce **cans** black
beans, undrained

1 14.5-ounce **can**
tomatoes

DIRECTIONS

1. In a non-stick pan, sauté the beef until brown over medium heat. Drain the excess oil.

2. Place all ingredients in a stock pot. Bring the soup to a boil then reduce to low heat and simmer for 10 minutes.

3. Serve the soup with the fat-free ranch dressing on top.

NUTRITION FACTS (PER SERVING)

CALORIES	108	KCal
PROTEIN	10.0	g
FAT	1.1	g
CARBOHYDRATES	14.6	g
SUGAR	1.4	g
SODIUM	268	mg

MAIN COURSE

BEEF AND BROCCOLI STIR FRY

PREP TIME

15 MINUTES

COOK TIME

15 MINUTES

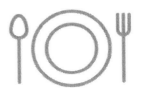

SERVES

6

INGREDENTS

Main Ingredients

12 ounces sirloin steak, visible fat trimmed, very thinly sliced against the grain

1 medium head broccoli, cut into florets

2 cloves garlic, minced

For beef marinade

1 teaspoon cornstarch

1 teaspoon low-sodium soy sauce

1/2 teaspoon sesame oil

1/8 teaspoon black pepper

For the sauce

2 teaspoons cornstarch

2 teaspoons stevia

1 1/2 teaspoons oyster-flavored sauce

1 teaspoons low-sodium soy sauce

1/2 teaspoon sesame oil

1/2 teaspoon Mirin, Chinese cooking wine or dry sherry

1/2 to 3/4 cup of water

DIRECTIONS

1. In a medium bowl, mix the sliced beef and all marinade ingredients together. Set aside for 15 minutes. In a small bowl, mix all sauce ingredients and stir until the cornstarch dissolve.

2. Over a pot, add 2-3 cups of water and bring it to a boil. Blanch the broccoli for at least 2 minutes. (Longer if you are in the first year post-surgery stage). Drain and immediately run cold water for 15 seconds. Set aside.

3. Spray some fat-free cooking spray on a non-stick pan and heat over high heat for 1 minutes. Then add the beef to the pan. Spread the slices on the pan and sear to brown, about 1-2 minutes. Flip the meat and add garlic. Sear for 1 minute.

4. Add the sauce and stir for 30 seconds continuously or until the sauce boils and thickens.

5. Toss in the broccoli and mix well. Taste the sauce and adjust seasoning if needed. Serve immediately.

MAIN COURSE
SKINNY BEEF STROGANOFF

PREP TIME
5 MINUTES

COOK TIME
25 MINUTES

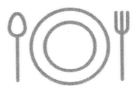

SERVES
8

INGREDENTS

1 pound 95% lean ground beef

1 7-ounce **package** Shirataki Fettuccini, rinsed and drained

8 ounces sliced mushrooms

1/4 cup chopped white onion

1 clove garlic, chopped

1 10.5-ounces **can** 98% fat-free cream of mushroom soup

1 1/2 cups fat-free half and half

2 tablespoons fat-free sour cream

3/4 teaspoon salt

1/4 teaspoon pepper

DIRECTIONS

1. In a large non-stick pan, Sauté the beef with onion and garlic until slightly brown over medium heat. Add mushroom and cook for about 5-10 minutes until mushroom are done.

2. Add the mushroom soup and half and half. Bring to a boil then reduce to low heat. Simmer for 15 minutes. Stir occasionally.

3. Add the drained Fettuccini and mix well. Cook for another 3-5 minutes. Serve immediately.

NUTRITION FACTS (PER SERVING)

CALORIES	141	KCal
PROTEIN	17.4	g
FAT	4.7	g
CARBOHYDRATES	6.9	g
SUGAR	2.5	g
SODIUM	394	mg

MAIN COURSE
ITALIAN-ESQUE
BEEF AND VEGGIE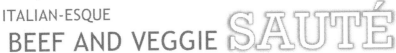

PREP TIME

15 MINUTES

COOK TIME

25 MINUTES

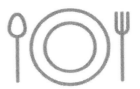

SERVES

8

INGREDENTS

1 **pound** round steak, cut into strips

1 medium zucchini, sliced into 1/4-inch pieces

1 medium yellow squash, sliced into 1/4-inch pieces

2 **cups** mushrooms, whole

2 **cups** 3 pepper & onion blend

1/2 **cup** no-sugar-added tomato and basil spaghetti sauce

1 **tablespoon** vinegar

1 **tablespoon** red wine

1 **teaspoon** salt

1 **teaspoon** Italian seasoning

Fat-free cooking spray

76

DIRECTIONS

1. In a large non-stick pan, Sauté the beef until brown over medium heat. Season with salt and Italian seasoning to taste. Set aside in a bowl.

2. Sauté the pepper/onion blend in the same pan until cooked through. Pour the mixture over the beef.

3. Sauté the mushrooms until cooked through. Drain the excess liquid then add meat, vegetables and all other ingredients. Mix well and bring to a boil. Then reduce to low heat, cover and simmer for 5-7 minutes. Serve immediately.

NUTRITION FACTS (PER SERVING)

CALORIES	117	KCal
PROTEIN	14.4	g
FAT	4.6	g
CARBOHYDRATES	4.5	g
SUGAR	2.4	g
SODIUM	458	mg

MAIN COURSE

MEATLOAF CUPCAKES
WITH MASHED CAULIFLOWER

PREP TIME

10 MINUTES

COOK TIME

40 MINUTES

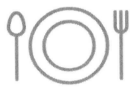

SERVES

12

INGREDENTS

For the Meatloaf Cupcakes:

1 1/4 pounds 93% lean ground beef

1 cup grated zucchini

1/2 cup seasoned breadcrumbs

1/4 cup low sugar/salt ketchup

2 tablespoons minced onion

1 large egg

1 teaspoon salt

For the Cauliflower Frosting:

1 medium head cauliflower, chopped

2 large garlic cloves, peeled and halved

2 tablespoons fat free sour cream

2 tablespoons fat-free chicken broth

1 tablespoon skim milk

1/2 tablespoon light butter

2 tablespoons fresh thyme

1/2 teaspoon salt

1/4 teaspoon pepper

DIRECTIONS

1. Put the cauliflower and garlic in a large pot with salt and enough water to cover; bring to a boil.

2. Cover and reduce heat; simmer for 5-10 minutes or until cauliflower are tender.

3. Drain and return cauliflower and garlic to pan.

4. Add sour cream and remaining ingredients. Using a masher or blender, mash the mixture until smooth. Season with salt and pepper.

5. Next, preheat the oven to 350°. Line a muffin tin with foil liners.

6. In a separate bowl or container, mix the turkey, zucchini, onion, breadcrumbs, ketchup, egg, and salt. Place meatloaf mixture into muffin tins filling them to the top. They should be flat at the top.

7. Bake uncovered for 18-20 minutes or until cooked well. Remove from tins and place onto a baking dish.

8. Pipe the "frosting" onto the meatloaf cupcakes and serve.

NUTRITION FACTS (PER SERVING)

CALORIES	172	KCal
PROTEIN	38.0	g
FAT	4.4	g
CARBOHYDRATES	12.5	g
SUGAR	4.3	g
SODIUM	346	mg

MAIN COURSE

GARDEN VEGETABLE BEEF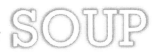

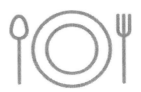

PREP TIME	COOK TIME	SERVES
10 MINUTES	40 MINUTES	4

INGREDENTS

1/2 **pound** 95% lean ground beef

3 **cups** fat-free beef broth

1 1/2 **cup** chopped cabbage

2/3 **cup** sliced carrots

1/2 **cup** diced onion

1/2 **cup** diced zucchini

1/2 **cup** frozen green beans

2 **cloves** garlic, minced

1 **tablespoon** tomato past

1/2 **teaspoon** dried basil

1/4 **teaspoon** dried oregano

1/4 **teaspoon** salt

DIRECTIONS

1. In a large non-stick pan, Sauté the beef until brown over medium heat. Drain excess fat.

2. Sauté carrots, onion and garlic over low heat for about 5 minutes until softened

3. Add beef, broth, cabbage, green beans, tomato paste and spice. Mix well, cover and simmer for 25 minutes.

4. Add in zucchini and cook for another 5 minutes

NUTRITION FACTS (PER SERVING)

CALORIES	122	KCal
PROTEIN	15.2	g
FAT	3.0	g
CARBOHYDRATES	8.7	g
SUGAR	4.0	g
SODIUM	510	mg

MAIN COURSE

BEEF STUFFED
ZUCCHINI BOAT

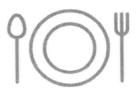

PREP TIME	COOK TIME	SERVES
10 MINUTES	50 MINUTES	4

INGREDENTS

2 medium zucchini, sliced in half

8 ounces 95% lean ground beef

1/2 cup finely chopped red bell pepper

1/2 cup finely chopped yellow bell pepper

1/4 cup finely chopped red onion

2 gloves garlic, minced

1/4 cup whole wheat breadcrumbs

1/4 cup no-added-sugar tomato sauce

1/4 cup low-fat parmesan cheese, grated and divided

1/4 teaspoon salt

1/8 teaspoon pepper

Fat-free cooking spray

82

DIRECTIONS

1. Pre-heat the over to 350°F.

2. In a non-stick pan, sauté the beef until brown over medium heat. Drain the excess oil and add to a large mixing bowl.

3. Slice the Zucchini along the long way. Scoop out the flesh to leave a 1/2-inch thick boat. Chop the scooped-out flesh and add to the mixing bowl.

4. Add in bell peppers, onion, garlic, breadcrumbs, tomato sauce, half of the parmesan cheese, salt and pepper. Mix well and fill the zucchini boats.

5. Place the zucchini boat into a baking dish and cover tightly with foil.

6. Bake for 45 minutes. Sprinkle the remaining cheese on top during the last 10 minutes.

NUTRITION FACTS (PER SERVING)

CALORIES	173	KCal
PROTEIN	18.2	g
FAT	4.8	g
CARBOHYDRATES	12.9	g
SUGAR	3.2	g
SODIUM	337	mg

MAIN COURSE

INDIAN
MADRAS CURRY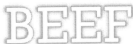

PREP TIME
15 MINUTES

COOK TIME
1 HOUR 45 MINUTES

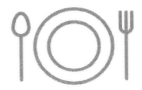

SERVES
10

INGREDENTS

Main ingredients

2 pounds round steak, diced

1 cup fat-free beef broth

1/4 cup tomato paste

1 tablespoon white vinegar

1 medium onion, diced

Non-fat cooking spray

For curry paste

2 cloves garlic, crushed

2 teaspoon crushed ginger

1/4 cup ground coriander

2 tablespoons ground cumin

1 teaspoon black mustard seeds

1 teaspoon chilli powder

1 teaspoon ground turmeric

1 teaspoon salt

DIRECTIONS

1. In a medium bowl, Combine all the ingredients for the curry paste. Add vinegar and 2 tablespoons of water and stir into a smooth consistency.

2. In a non-stick pan, sauté the onion over medium heat until softened. Add in the paste, stir and cook until the onion falls apart.

3. Add the meat, tomato paste and stock. Stir and bring the mixture to a boil then reduce to low heat. Cover and simmer for 1 hour 30 minutes

NUTRITION FACTS (PER SERVING)

CALORIES	160	KCal
PROTEIN	24.3	g
FAT	4.8	g
CARBOHYDRATES	4.9	g
SUGAR	1.0	g
SODIUM	389	mg

MAIN COURSE

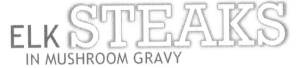

ELK STEAKS
IN MUSHROOM GRAVY

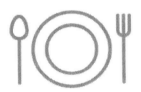

PREP TIME	COOK TIME	SERVES
5 MINUTES	5 HOURS 25 MINUES	24

INGREDENTS

4 pounds ELK steaks

3 10.5-ounce cans 98% fat-free cream of mushroom soup

4 cups sliced mushroom

3 cups skim milk

1 cup fat-free sour cream

1/4 cup corn starch

3 teaspoon salt

DIRECTIONS

1. Brown the steaks over a grill/griddle/pan. Transfer t0 the slow cooker and put the mushroom on top.

2. In a large bowl, combine soup, milk and salt to taste. Cover and cook on high for 4 hours

3. In a small bowl, dissolve the corn starch into 1 tablespoon of water. Add into the mixture and stir well. Cook for another hour or until meat is tender.

4. Pour in sour cream and serve.

MAIN COURSE

SLOW COOKED
ROUND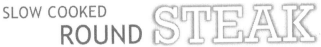

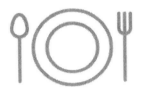

PREP TIME	COOK TIME	SERVES
15 MINUTES	6 HOURS 15 MINUTES	14

INGREDENTS

2 **pounds** round steak

4 small potatoes, peeled and cut into quarters

2 **stocks** celery, chopped

1 **cup** baby carrots

1 10.5-ounces **can** Beef broth

2 **cups** water

2 **cloves** garlic

DIRECTIONS

1. Combine all the ingredients into a crockpot.

2. Depending on the crock pot, cook for 5 to 6 hours. Faster crock pots will cook this dish faster.

3. Remove from crock pot and serve.

NUTRITION FACTS (PER SERVING)

CALORIES	142	KCal
PROTEIN	15.8	g
FAT	4.8	g
CARBOHYDRATES	8.5	g
SUGAR	0.9	g
SODIUM	205	mg

MAIN COURSE

SKINNY BOLOGNESE SAUCE

PREP TIME

30 MINUTES

COOK TIME

6 HOURS

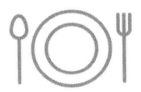

SERVES

8

INGREDENTS

1 pound 93% lean ground beef

1 1/2 28-ounces **can** whole-peeled tomatoes

1 cup chopped onion

1 clove garlic

2 tablespoons black pepper

1 tablespoon oregano

1 tablespoon dried basil leaves

1 tablespoon grated parmesan cheese

1 teaspoon Italian seasoning

1 teaspoon salt

1 teaspoon sugar

1/2 teaspoon onion powder

1/2 teaspoon garlic powder

DIRECTIONS

1. Blend the tomatoes into a smooth consistency. Add the tomatoes, garlic, half of the black pepper, oregano, basil, cheese, Italian seasoning, salt, sugar, onion powder, garlic powder and 3/4 of the onion into the slow cooker.

2. Brown the meat with the remaining black pepper and onion. Then add to the slow cooker. Stir well.

3. Cook the sauce on low for 5-6 hours.

NUTRITION FACTS (PER SERVING)

CALORIES	138	KCal
PROTEIN	14.1	g
FAT	4.4	g
CARBOHYDRATES	10.4	g
SUGAR	4.5	g
SODIUM	575	mg

MAIN COURSE

SOUTHWEST BEEF

WITH GRILLED PEPPERS

PREP TIME

6 HOURS

COOK TIME

30 MINUTES

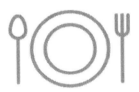

SERVES

6

INGREDENTS

Main Ingredients

1 1/2 pounds round steak, cut into 1-inch thick

1 red bell pepper, quartered

1 yellow bell pepper, quartered

1 green bell pepper, quartered

1 dash of salt

For the beef marinade

1/2 cup fat-free Italian dressing

2 tablespoons lime juice

1/2 tablespoon honey

1 1/2 teaspoons ground cumin

DIRECTIONS

1. In a small bowl, combine all ingredients for the marinade and mix well.

2. In a large resealable bag, add the steak and 1/3 cup of the marinade. Mix well and marinade overnight. Refrigerate the remaining marinade.

3. Scrap off excess marinade and discard the used marinade. Brush the bell peppers with some of the remaining marinade.

4. Place the steak and peppers on the grill. Grill the steak for 16-18 minutes and 12-15 minutes for the peppers. Turning and brushing the steak with the remaining marinade occasionally until 5 minutes before it is done.

5. Thinly slice the steak and season with salt. Serve with bell peppers immediately.

NUTRITION FACTS (PER SERVING)

CALORIES	176	KCal
PROTEIN	27.1	g
FAT	4.1	g
CARBOHYDRATES	7.7	g
SUGAR	4.7	g
SODIUM	205	mg

MAIN COURSE

CHINESE
PORK AND CELERY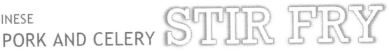

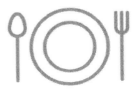

PREP TIME
10 MINUTES

COOK TIME
20 MINUTES

SERVES
8

INGREDENTS

14 ounces lean boneless pork, visible fat removed, thinly sliced

4 stalks celery, sliced

6 spring onions, chopped

3 tomatoes, cut into wedges

4 ounces fat-free beef stock

1 clove garlic

1 tablespoon low-sodium soy sauce

2 teaspoons corn starch

1 teaspoon olive oil

1 teaspoon grated ginger

DIRECTIONS

1. In a small bowl, mix the soy sauce and corn starch. Add stock and set aside.

2. Add the oil in wok or non-stick pan over high heat. Add ginger and garlic and cook for 30 second. Add the celery and onions and sauté briefly until slightly softened. Remove the vegetables.

3. Sauté the pork until brown. Add sauce and cook until thickened. Stir continuously. Add vegetables and tomatoes and stir well. Cover and heat for 1 minutes. Serve immediately.

NUTRITION FACTS (PER SERVING)

CALORIES	83	KCal
PROTEIN	12.5	g
FAT	1.9	g
CARBOHYDRATES	3.8	g
SUGAR	1.7	g
SODIUM	290	mg

MAIN COURSE

GARLIC LIME
MARINATED **PORK CHOPS**

PREP TIME
20 MINUTES

COOK TIME
10 MINUTES

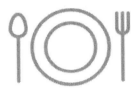

SERVES
8

INGREDENTS

4 (6-ounces each) lean boneless pork chops

4 **cloves** garlic, crushed

1 **teaspoon** kosher salt

1 **teaspoon** lime zest

1/2 **teaspoon** pepper

1/2 **teaspoon** cumin

1/2 **teaspoon** paprika

1/2 **teaspoon** chilli powder

1/2 lime, juice only

DIRECTIONS

1. In a large bowl, mix all ingredient and stir well. Refrigerate for at least 20 minutes to marinate.

2. Preheat the oven and set it to broiler

3. Line broiler with foil and place the pork on top. Broil for 4-5 minutes for each side or until brown

NUTRITION FACTS (PER SERVING)

CALORIES	112	KCal
PROTEIN	19.0	g
FAT	3.0	g
CARBOHYDRATES	0.9	g
SUGAR	1.7	g
SODIUM	184	mg

MAIN COURSE

MEGA PORK MEATBALLS

PREP TIME
10 MINUTES

COOK TIME
35 MINUTES

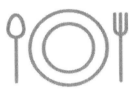

SERVES
8

INGREDENTS

1 pound extra lean ground pork

1 egg

1/2 cup whole wheat breadcrumbs, crushed

1/4 cup low sugar/salt ketchup

3 tablespoon stevia (brown sugar blend)

1 tablespoon onion flakes

1 teaspoon dry mustard

1/2 teaspoon salt

1/4 teaspoon ground pepper

Fat-free cooking spray

DIRECTIONS

1. Preheat the oven to 375°F

2. In a small bowl, mix ketchup, stevia and dry mustard. In a large bowl, combine pork, onion flakes, breadcrumbs, salt, pepper, egg and 2 tablespoons of the ketchup mixture.

3. Spray muffin tin with fat-free cooking spray. Divide the meat under 8 portions and roll into balls. Brush the remaining ketchup mixture on top of each meatball.

4. Bake for 30 minutes or until brown.

NUTRITION FACTS (PER SERVING)

CALORIES	129	KCal
PROTEIN	13.1	g
FAT	3.8	g
CARBOHYDRATES	11.1	g
SUGAR	3.0	g
SODIUM	279	mg

MAIN COURSE
CRUSTLESS QUICHE

PREP TIME

10 MINUTES

COOK TIME

50 MINUTES

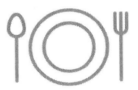

SERVES

6

INGREDENTS

1 **cup** fat-free cottage cheese

2 **cups** liquid egg substitute

1/2 **cup** broccoli, blanched and chopped

1/2 **cup** 5% fat ham, diced

1/2 **cup** low fat cheddar cheese, shredded

Salt and pepper to taste

Fat free cooking spray

DIRECTIONS

1. Preheat the oven to 375°F

2. In a large bowl, combine all ingredients.

3. Spray pie dish with fat-free cooking spray.
   Add the mixture to the dish and spread
   evenly.

4. Bake for about 45 minutes or until cooked
   through.

NUTRITION FACTS (PER SERVING)

CALORIES	107	KCal
PROTEIN	18.7	g
FAT	1.4	g
CARBOHYDRATES	4.5	g
SUGAR	1.2	g
SODIUM	514	mg

MAIN COURSE
BEER GRILLED PORK CHOPS

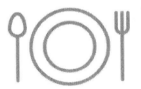

PREP TIME	COOK TIME	SERVES
4 HOURS	30 MINUTES	8

INGREDENTS

4 (6-ounces each) extra lean boneless pork chops

1 cup beer

1/4 cup low-sodium soy sauce

2 tablespoons stevia (brown sugar blend)

2 teaspoons grated ginger roots

DIRECTIONS

1. In a large resalable bag, add all ingredients and seal the bag. Turn and spread the marinade evenly. Refrigerate for 4 hours

2. Prepare the kettle-style grill with medium hot coal. Scrap off the marinade from the pork chops.

3. Place the chops on the grill. Cover grill and heat for 5 minutes then flip the chops and heat for another 5 minutes.

NUTRITION FACTS (PER SERVING)

CALORIES	131	KCal
PROTEIN	17.8	g
FAT	3.0	g
CARBOHYDRATES	5.3	g
SUGAR	2.0	g
SODIUM	265	mg

MAIN COURSE
SKINNY CHALUPA

PREP TIME

5 MINUTES

COOK TIME

10 HOURS

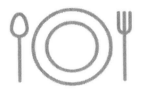

SERVES

22

INGREDENTS

3 **pounds** extra lean pork roast

1 **pound** dry pinto beans

1 4-ounces **can** chopped green chillies

2 **cloves** garlic, minced

2 **tablespoons** chilli powder

1 **tablespoon** ground cumin

1 **tablespoon** dried oregano

1/2 **tablespoon** salt

DIRECTIONS

1. Place the beans in the slow cooker and add water until its half an inch above the bean. Cook on high for 1 hour and leave it to sit overnight.

2. Take out the bean with the water. Put the roast in the bottom of the cooker then return the beans and add all other ingredients to the pot. Add water to cover all ingredients.

3. Cook on high for 1 hour then reduce to low and cook for 6 hours.

4. Take out the meat and shred it with forks. Return the shredded meat to the cooker and cook on high for 1 more hour.

NUTRITION FACTS (PER SERVING)

CALORIES	124	KCal
PROTEIN	11.0	g
FAT	3.0	g
CARBOHYDRATES	14.0	g
SUGAR	0.7	g
SODIUM	184	mg

MAIN COURSE
LIME MUSTARD LAMB CHOPS

PREP TIME
15 MINUTES

COOK TIME
15 MINUTES

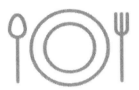

SERVES
4

INGREDENTS

4 (4-ounces each) lean lamp chops

1 **clove** garlic, minced

2 **tablespoons** lemon juice

2 **tablespoons** parsley

2 **tablespoons** brown mustard

1 **teaspoon** lemon zest

1/2 **teaspoon** rosemary

DIRECTIONS

1. Preheat the broiler.

2. Cover the lamp chop with lemon juice and set aside for 15 minutes. In a small bowl, mix the remaining ingredients.

3. Spray the pan and place the chop. Spread half of the sauce on top.

4. Broil for about 4-5 minutes. Flip and spread the remaining sauce on top. Broil for another 4-5 minutes.

NUTRITION FACTS (PER SERVING)

CALORIES	115	KCal
PROTEIN	17.5	g
FAT	4.2	g
CARBOHYDRATES	0.6	g
SUGAR	0.0	g
SODIUM	55	mg

MAIN COURSE
DIJON AND HERBS **LAMB CHOPS**

PREP TIME
10 MINUTES

COOK TIME
20 MINUTES

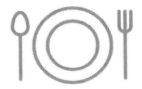

SERVES
3

INGREDENTS

3 (4-ounces each) lean lamp chops

1 tablespoon Dijon Mustard

2 tablespoons chopped parsley

2 tablespoons chopped rosemary

1 tablespoon oregano, crumbled

1/2 teaspoon salt

1/4 teaspoon pepper

DIRECTIONS

1. Preheat the oven to 375°F.

2. Spread out the herbs on a large plate. Cover the lamp chop with mustard evenly. Coat the lamp chops in herbs.

3. Roast for about 15-20 minutes

NUTRITION FACTS (PER SERVING)

CALORIES	134	KCal
PROTEIN	18.6	g
FAT	4.6	g
CARBOHYDRATES	1.2	g
SUGAR	0.1	g
SODIUM	320	mg

MAIN COURSE
LAMB ROGAN JOSH

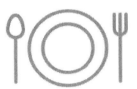

PREP TIME	COOK TIME	SERVES
5 MINUTES	45 MINUTES	8

INGREDENTS

1 pound leg of lamb, visible fat removed, cubed

1 package 12-ounces frozen soup vegetables

1 15-ounces **jar** Patak's Rogan Josh sauce

Fat-free cooking spray

DIRECTIONS

1. Sauté lamb in large non-stick pan until brown over medium heat.

2. Add all ingredients and 2 cups of water to the pan. Bring it to a boil then reduce to low heat. Simmer for about 45 minutes.

NUTRITION FACTS (PER SERVING)

CALORIES	138	KCal
PROTEIN	13.5	g
FAT	4.9	g
CARBOHYDRATES	10.0	g
SUGAR	2.6	g
SODIUM	369	mg

MAIN COURSE
SPICY LAMB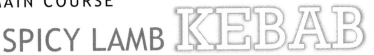

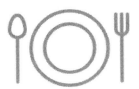

PREP TIME

3 HOURS

COOK TIME

30 MINUTES

SERVES

8

INGREDENTS

1 **pound** boneless leg of lamb, trimmed and cubed

1 **cup** fat-free plain yogurt

2 **cloves** garlic, minced

2 **tablespoons** lemon juice

1 1/2 **tablespoons** grated ginger

1 **tablespoon** grated lemon rind

2 **teaspoons** paprika

1 1/2 **teaspoons** salt

1 **teaspoon** ground coriander

1 **teaspoon** ground cumin

1/2 **teaspoon** freshly ground black pepper

1/4 **teaspoon** ground red pepper

DIRECTIONS

1. In a large resalable bag, add all ingredients and seal the bag. Turn and spread the marinade evenly. Refrigerate for 3 hours

2. Remove the lamb and divide into 8 portions. Thread onto 10-inch skewers.

3. Grill the lamb for 8 minutes. Turn occasionally.

NUTRITION FACTS (PER SERVING)

CALORIES	85	KCal
PROTEIN	14.0	g
FAT	2.4	g
CARBOHYDRATES	1.3	g
SUGAR	0.9	g
SODIUM	44	mg

MAIN COURSE
CLASSIC LAMB STEW

PREP TIME
30 MINUTES

COOK TIME
8 HOURS

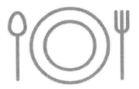

SERVES
8

INGREDENTS

1 **pound** lean lamb meat, cubed

2 medium **stalks** celery, chopped

2 **cups** diced potatoes

1 **cup** chopped carrots

1 **cup** frozen pea

1/4 **cup** chopped onion

8 **ounces** red wine

1 **tablespoon** rosemary

1 **teaspoon** thyme

Fat-free cooking spray

114

DIRECTIONS

1. Brown the lamb cube over medium heat. Transfer the lamb to slow cooker. Add the wine to deglaze pan and add to slow cooker.

2. Add all ingredients into slow cooker.

3. Cook on low for 6-8 hours

NUTRITION FACTS (PER SERVING)

CALORIES	174	KCal
PROTEIN	13.6	g
FAT	4.9	g
CARBOHYDRATES	13.2	g
SUGAR	2.3	g
SODIUM	87	mg

MAIN COURSE

BRAISED LAMB SHANKS

WITH WHITE BEANS

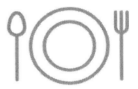

PREP TIME

30 MINUTES

COOK TIME

8 HOURS

SERVES

6

INGREDENTS

2 8-ounces lamb shanks

1 **cup** dry white beans

1 medium onion, coarsely diced

6 **cloves** garlic, peeled and halved

1 **teaspoon** salt

1 **teaspoon** black pepper

DIRECTIONS

1. Preheat the oven to 375°F.

2. Put the shanks in a heavy baking pan and cover with onion and garlic. Bake for about 45-60 minutes or until brown.

3. Put the shank in slow cooker, add beans and enough water to cover all ingredients by about 1 inch

4. Cook on high until boiling then reduce to low.

5. Cook for 6 to 8 hours or until beans are tender.

NUTRITION FACTS (PER SERVING)

CALORIES	160	KCal
PROTEIN	19.2	g
FAT	3.4	g
CARBOHYDRATES	12.9	g
SUGAR	0.0	g
SODIUM	440	mg

MAIN COURSE

SHRIMP SCAMPI

PREP TIME
5 MINUTES

COOK TIME
10 MINUTES

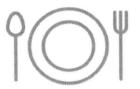

SERVES
4

INGREDENTS

3/4 **Pound** uncooked shrimp, peeled

3/4 **Tablespoon** olive oil

1 medium green onion, diced

1 **tablespoon** lemon juice

1 **tablespoon** Parmesan cheese

3/4 **teaspoon** parsley

1/2 **teaspoon** basil

1/2 **teaspoon** salt

1/4 **teaspoon** garlic powder

DIRECTIONS

1. In a medium skillet, heat oil over medium high heat.

2. Add shrimp and other ingredients. Cook 3-7 minutes depending on the size of shrimp.

3. Remove from heat; sprinkle with Parmesan cheese.

NUTRITION FACTS (PER SERVING)

CALORIES	124	KCal
PROTEIN	18.1	g
FAT	4.5	g
CARBOHYDRATES	2.0	g
SUGAR	0.1	g
SODIUM	310	mg

MAIN COURSE

TUNA
~~SHRIMP~~ AND SHIRATAKI FETTUCINE

PREP TIME
5 MINUTES

COOK TIME
20 MINUTES

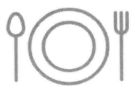
SERVES
6

INGREDENTS

I can Tuna fish
~~1 pound peeled shrimp~~

8 ounces Shirataki
Fettuccine noodles

1/2 cup white wine

1 tablespoon crushed red
peppers
Kids didn't like
substitute with other
flavor next time
i. e. onion &garlic or italian flavorings.

1 1/2 tablespoons Extra
Virgin Olive Oil

2 teaspoon minced garlic

~~1/2 teaspoon salt~~ *Not needed*

1/4 teaspoon pepper

DIRECTIONS

1. Drain Shirataki noodles. Rinse noodles under cool water. Drain and squeeze out excess water as much as possible.

2. In a non-stick skillet, mix the shrimp, oil, pepper, and garlic. Cook until shrimp is pink. Make sure the shrimp is not overcooked or hardened.

3. During the last two minutes of cooking time, add the wine and let evaporate.

4. Toss shrimp mixture with noodles and serve.

NUTRITION FACTS (PER SERVING)

CALORIES	158	KCal
PROTEIN	15.7	g
FAT	4.9	g
CARBOHYDRATES	3.0	g
SUGAR	0.0	g
SODIUM	198	mg

MAIN COURSE

LEMON-DILL
GRILLED SHRIMPS

PREP TIME
20 MINUTES

COOK TIME
5 MINUTES

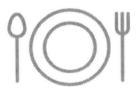

SERVES
4

INGREDENTS

1 **pound** shrimp, shelled and deveined

1/3 cup minced fresh dill

1/4 cup fresh lemon juice

1/2 tablespoon olive oil

4 teaspoons Dijon mustard

1/4 teaspoon salt

1/4 teaspoon black pepper

1 **clove** garlic, minced

Fat-free cooking spray

DIRECTIONS

1. Combine all the ingredients except for the cooking spray in a large zip-top plastic bag; seal and let marinate in refrigerator for about 20 minutes.

2. Remove shrimp from bag, and dispose of marinade.

3. Prepare grill or broiler.

4. Place shrimp on a grill rack or broiler pan coated with cooking spray. Cook over medium heat for 2-3 minutes on each side or until the shrimp is pink and well-cooked.

NUTRITION FACTS (PER SERVING)

CALORIES	163	KCal
PROTEIN	33.0	g
FAT	3.4	g
CARBOHYDRATES	3.0	g
SUGAR	<1	g
SODIUM	434	mg

MAIN COURSE

CRISPY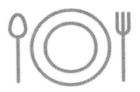

WITH JAPANESE COCKTAIL SAUCE

PREP TIME	COOK TIME	SERVES
5 MINUTES	20 MINUTES	4

INGREDENTS

Main Ingredients

1 pound shrimp, peeled and deveined

1/2 cup panko breadcrumbs

1/4 cup white whole wheat flour

1/4 teaspoon paprika

2 tablespoons egg whites

For the Sauce

2 cups fresh spinach

1/2 cup shelled edamame

1/2 teaspoon wasabi paste

1/2 lemon, juiced

DIRECTIONS

1. Preheat the oven to 400 degrees.
2. Place the flour and paprika in one flat dish, the egg whites in a separate dish, and the panko in a resealable bag.
3. Place the shrimp in the flour and coat well, then place them in the egg whites. Next, place the shrimp into the bag of panko and shake well. Place the shrimp on the rack. Repeat with the remaining shrimp. Once all the shrimp have been breaded, coat them with non-stick cooking spray.
4. Bake 12-14 minutes, until the crust is slightly browned.
5. While baking the shrimp, prepare the sauce. Simmer the edamame in 2 cups of water for approximately 10 minutes, then add the spinach and cook 1 minute.
6. Drain the water, reserving one cup. Pour cold water over the edamame and spinach. Place the vegetables in a small food processor of blender with half of the reserved cup of cooking liquid. Pulse several times then add the wasabi and lemon juice and process until smooth.

NUTRITION FACTS (PER SERVING)

CALORIES	156	KCal
PROTEIN	33.9	g
FAT	1.4	g
CARBOHYDRATES	13.5	g
SUGAR	0.9	g
SODIUM	560	mg

MAIN COURSE
SHRIMP CEVICHE

PREP TIME

15 MINUTES

COOK TIME

10 MINUTES

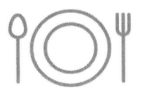

SERVES

4

INGREDENTS

1 pound medium raw shrimp, shelled and deveined

1 cup lime juice

4 medium tomatoes diced

1 small red onion, peeled and chopped

1 bunch cilantro, stemmed and chopped

2 serrano chili peppers, ribs and seeds removed, minced

DIRECTIONS

1. In a bowl, mix the shrimp and lime juice.

2. Cover and let sit for about 10 to 15 minutes or until the color turns to pink. Do not marinate too long, as the shrimp will "overcook" and harden.

3. Add the onions, tomatoes, chili peppers and cilantro.

4. Gently stir to combine.

5. Season with salt and serve cold.

NUTRITION FACTS (PER SERVING)

CALORIES	160	KCal
PROTEIN	25.0	g
FAT	1.0	g
CARBOHYDRATES	13.0	g
SUGAR	4.9	g
SODIUM	265	mg

MAIN COURSE

SHRIMP JAMBALAYA

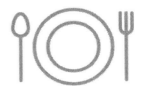

PREP TIME

5 MINUTES

COOK TIME

9 HOURS

SERVES

8

INGREDENTS

3/4 **pound** medium shrimp, raw, peeled and deveined

28 **ounces** canned tomatoes (undrained)

1 **cup** chopped onion

1 **cup** chopped green bell peppers

1 **cup** chopped celery

2 **cloves** chopped garlic

1 **cup** chopped smoked sausage

1 **tablespoon** dried parsley

1/2 **teaspoon** dried thyme

1/2 **teaspoon** salt

1/4 **teaspoon** pepper

1/4 **teaspoon** Tabasco sauce

DIRECTIONS

1. Add all ingredients except for the shrimp into a 3-6 quart slow cooker.

2. Cover & cook on low heat for approximately 7-8 hours (or on high for 3-4 hours).

3. Add in the cleaned shrimp, cover & cook on low heat for about 1 hour or until shrimp are pink, firm and well-cooked.

NUTRITION FACTS (PER SERVING)

CALORIES	113	KCal
PROTEIN	15.0	g
FAT	4.2	g
CARBOHYDRATES	7.5	g
SUGAR	4.2	g
SODIUM	501	mg

MAIN COURSE
CREAMY CURRY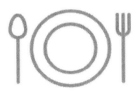

PREP TIME

5 MINUTES

COOK TIME

15 MINUTES

SERVES

2

INGREDENTS

1 package 12.3-ounces lite-firm silken tofu

1 cup snapped green beans

1/4 cup chopped carrots

2 tablespoons low-fat sour cream

1 tablespoon curry sauce

1 tablespoon dried cilantro

Fat-free cooking spray

DIRECTIONS

1. Spray the pan then add curry sauce. Heat over medium heat for 30 seconds.

2. Add tofu, green beans, carrots and cilantro. Heat and stir until cooked to desired texture. Then add sour cream, stir well and serve.

NUTRITION FACTS (PER SERVING)

CALORIES	139	KCal
PROTEIN	13.0	g
FAT	4.9	g
CARBOHYDRATES	11.8	g
SUGAR	1.6	g
SODIUM	363	mg

MAIN COURSE
SKINNY MOZZARELLA STICKS

PREP TIME

5 MINUTES

COOK TIME

25 MINUTES

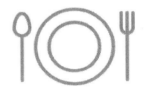

SERVES

12

INGREDENTS

1 package 12-ounces 2% low-fat Mozzarella string cheese

1 large egg

1/2 cup whole wheat breadcrumbs

1 teaspoon Italian seasoning

Fat-free cooking spray

DIRECTIONS

1. Put the rack in upper third position and preheat the oven to 350°F .

2. Line a baking sheet with foil and grease it slightly

3. Whisk egg for 5 minutes or until foamy. Heat Italian seasoning with breadcrumbs until slightly brown over medium heat. Spread the breadcrumbs on a large plate.

4. Dip the cheese in the egg then coat with breadcrumbs. Place on the baking sheet.

5. Bake 5-6 minutes. Serve immediately.

NUTRITION FACTS (PER SERVING)

CALORIES	93	KCal
PROTEIN	9.0	g
FAT	4.8	g
CARBOHYDRATES	4.1	g
SUGAR	1.0	g
SODIUM	243	mg

MAIN COURSE
SOUTHWEST TOFU SCRAMBLE

PREP TIME
15 MINUTES

COOK TIME
15 MINUTES

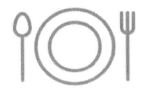

SERVES
2

INGREDENTS

8 ounces extra firm tofu

2 cups kale, loosely chopped

1/2 red pepper, thinly sliced

1/4 red onion, thinly sliced

1/2 teaspoon sea salt

1/2 teaspoon garlic powder

1/2 teaspoon cumin powder

1/4 teaspoon chilli powder

1/4 teaspoon turmeric

Fat-free cooking spray

DIRECTIONS

1. Roll the tofu in a clean towel and place a heavy subject on top for 15 minutes.

2. In a small bowl, mix the spice with 2 tablespoons of water.

3. Sauté the onion and bell peppers over medium heat until softened. Add kale and cover for 2 minutes. Season with salt and pepper.

4. Put the tofu into 1-inch cube.

5. Move the veggie to the side. Add the tofu and sauté for 2 minutes. Then add 3/4 of the sauce over the tofu and the remaining over the veggie. Mix well and cook for another 5-7 minutes.

NUTRITION FACTS (PER SERVING)

CALORIES	103	KCal
PROTEIN	10.7	g
FAT	2.2	g
CARBOHYDRATES	8.7	g
SUGAR	0.2	g
SODIUM	95	mg

MAIN COURSE
TOFU NOODLES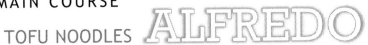

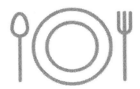

PREP TIME
5 MINUTES

COOK TIME
25 MINUTES

SERVES
2

INGREDENTS

1 **pack** 4-ounces Shirataki Tofu Fettuccine, rinsed, drained and cut into pieces

2 **cups** broccoli

1 5-ounces **can** chunk light tuna in water, drained

1 **cup** Walden Farms Alfredo Dressing

1 **cup** sliced zucchini

1 **ounce** low-fat blue cheese

1 **tablespoon** basil

1 **teaspoon** garlic

Salt to taste

136

DIRECTIONS

1. In a small bowl, mix tuna, garlic, basil, alfredo dressing and set aside.

2. Sauté the broccoli over low heat for 5 minutes then add the zucchini and cook for about 3 minutes. Set aside.

3. Heat the noodle over low heat for about 2 minutes. Add the tuna sauce and put on medium heat until simmering. Add the vegetables and cook for another 1-2 minutes.

4. Reduce to low heat and add the blue cheese. Serve once the cheese melts.

NUTRITION FACTS (PER SERVING)

CALORIES	144	KCal
PROTEIN	23.4	g
FAT	4.7	g
CARBOHYDRATES	12.5	g
SUGAR	1.6	g
SODIUM	502	mg

MAIN COURSE

VEGGIE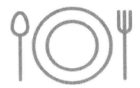

PREP TIME	COOK TIME	SERVES
10 MINUTES	45 MINUTES	8

INGREDENTS

1 12-ounces **package** vegetarian burger crumbles

1 -ounce **packet** 1 beef and onion dry soup mix

1/2 cup whole wheat breadcrumbs, crushed

2 large eggs, beaten

1 1/2 teaspoon olive oil

1/2 teaspoon garlic powder

Salt and pepper to taste

Fat-free cooking spray

DIRECTIONS

1. Preheat the oven to 400°F.

2. Spray a 9X5 loaf pan. In a large bowl, combine all ingredients until well incorporated.

3. Pour the mixture into the pan and spread evenly.

4. Bake 30-45 minutes until firm.

NUTRITION FACTS (PER SERVING)

CALORIES	125	KCal
PROTEIN	10.4	g
FAT	4.6	g
CARBOHYDRATES	10.2	g
SUGAR	1.6	g
SODIUM	496	mg

MAIN COURSE

GREEN BEAN AND
WISCONSIN CHEESE CASSEROLE

PREP TIME

15 MINUTES

COOK TIME

1 HOUR 15 MINUTES

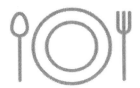

SERVES

10

INGREDENTS

2 pounds fresh whole green beans, trimmed and steamed

1/2 pound sliced mushroom

2 1/4 cups fat-free milk, divided

1/4 cup whole wheat flour

1 yellow onion, sliced into thin rings

2 cups low-fat swiss cheese

5 tablespoons of light buttery spread

Salt and pepper to taste

DIRECTIONS

1. Preheat the oven to 375°F.

2. Sauté mushroom in 2 tablespoons of buttery spread over medium-high heat until golden brown. Set aside.

3. Heat the remaining buttery spread with flour and stir continuously for 1 minute. Add milk and cook for about 5 minutes until silky.

4. Remove from heat and add 1 1/2 cup of cheese in batch. Stir until melted and season with salt and pepper.

5. In a large bowl, mix green beans, mushroom and cheese sauce. Pour into a 9 x 13 casserole dish and top with the remaining cheese.

6. Bake for 40 minutes.

NUTRITION FACTS (PER SERVING)

CALORIES	114	KCal
PROTEIN	7.6	g
FAT	3.6	g
CARBOHYDRATES	20.2	g
SUGAR	2.8	g
SODIUM	347	mg

It's A Total Effort

As already mentioned in past chapters, gastric sleeve surgery is just a part of the journey towards your ideal weight. After you have recovered from the surgical operation, you have your work cut out for you in terms of better food choices, a more active lifestyle, and overall positive outlook that will transform your health and wellness. It's a lot of changes that you will have to get used to, but if you persevere and stick it out, it will be worth all the effort.

Take the case of Tina Tait, a sleeve gastrectomy patient at Piedmont Atlanta Hospital in Georgia. She was physically active and a regular participant in 5K runs and fundraising walks for breast cancer research, but somehow she still found it very difficult to lose weight. Before her surgical procedure, she weighed about 250 pounds.

"That was just the most helpless feeling in the world – there's nothing else I could have done that would have made me more successful," Tait said. "There's just nothing like that frustration."

Tait did not have diabetes or other conditions known as co-morbidites, so her doctor recommended that she undergo gastric sleeve surgery instead of gastric bypass or adjustable gastric band. Her physician also suggested this procedure because it would have the fastest recovery time.

Tait recalled, "After the surgery, I woke up in the hospital bed and felt like I had just had a vigorous Pilates workout. My abs were tight – I was almost unconvinced that anything had been done. I felt satisfaction for the first time in my life."

Also, Tait is quick to point out that unlike many people's misconception, weight loss surgery is not the easy way out.

"Some people say it's the easy way out and it's definitely not," she says. "[The surgery] doesn't keep you from eating things you're not supposed to eat. You still have to control what you put in your body."

Now, Tait has lost 120 pounds and weighs 130 pounds. She remains committed to the healthy lifestyle by eating right and staying active. In fact, she recently completed her first marathon.

Thank You for Reading!

Thank you very much for downloading this eBook and for going through the information we presented!

We realize that you have probably spent a lot of time looking elsewhere for information related to your weight loss goals, whether it is the Internet, books, magazines, newspapers, or other sources. We appreciate that you took the time to read what we have to say.

Get a BONUS gift exclusive to my readers for FREE!

☐ *A4-sized printable **Complete Food List Poster** for fluid and puree stages*
☐ *A4-sized printable Daily **Dietary Reminders Posters** for all post-surgery stages*

☐ ***Scan the QR code and get yours now!***

Made in the USA
Middletown, DE
06 May 2017